T0100423

Invasive Fungal Rhinosinusitis

Gauri Mankekar

Editor

Invasive Fungal
Rhinosinusitis

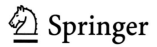 Springer

Editor
Gauri Mankekar
ENT, PD Hinduja Hospital
Mumbai
India

ISBN 978-81-322-1529-5   ISBN 978-81-322-1530-1   (eBook)
DOI 10.1007/978-81-322-1530-1
Springer New Delhi Heidelberg New York Dordrecht London

Library of Congress Control Number: 2013948761

Springer is part of Springer Science+Business Media (www.springer.com)

Foreword

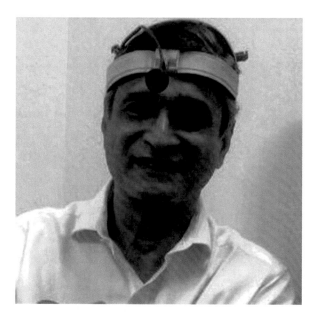

The incidence of invasive fungal sinusitis has seen a steep rise in recent years. It is commonly seen in immunocompromised patients. However, more and more cases are being seen in patients without obvious immunodeficiency, which is an alarming trend. Allergic fungal sinusitis is an entity that the nasal endoscopist encounters frequently while dealing with sinonasal polyposis, and surgery remains the mainstay of management. There is, however, divided opinion on whether these patients merit antifungal treatment. Invasive fungal sinusitis, on the other hand, is treated with antifungal drugs complemented by aggressive surgical debridement. Dr. Gauri Mankekar, who is a general otolaryngologist, has for several years focused her attention on the problem of invasive fungal sinusitis and has therefore gained immense experience in managing these patients both surgically and medically. This book is a result of this experience and deals with the subject in a very comprehensive manner. Starting with a very systematic classification, the book gives a very clear picture of the variety of presentations and diagnosis of fungal sinusitis.

The chapters on microbiology, pathology and radiology have been dealt with by experts in their respective fields in a very succinct manner. The medical management has been exhaustively covered so that the reader has complete information on the subject. The inclusion of "case studies" has been a very relevant and informative addition. This book will be of great value and is a "must read" for both the postgraduate student and the practicing clinician. Dr. Gauri Mankekar deserves to be complimented on her dedicated effort in bringing out this book.

Mumbai, India   Dr. M.V. Kirtane, MS (ENT)

Preface

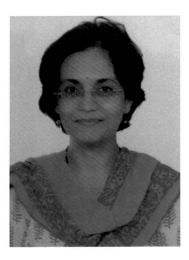

Dr. Gauri Mankekar

Several years ago I encountered my first paediatric patient of mucormycosis. The child had juvenile diabetes with ketoacidosis. The surgical treatment paradigm then was "aggressive debridement". It was indeed challenging to be "aggressive" with this small child, and I followed a "conservative approach" – restricting to repeated endoscopic debridement without orbital exenteration or palatal removal. Like most clinicians in such situations, there was the dilemma, then, whether "conservative" was the best approach. Luckily the child responded to treatment and I got interested in the management of invasive fungal sinusitis, but there wasn't a single comprehensive book on the subject – only several hundred published papers. This led to the idea of writing this book.

This book attempts to provide comprehensive information on invasive fungal sinusitis, the controversies regarding classification as well as its management. My colleagues from microbiology, pathology and radiology have provided an insight into the diagnostic aspects of the disease, while Dr. Soman, the infectious disease specialist, has provided a succinct chapter on medical management which forms the mainstay of the treatment. The chapter on case studies was included to sensitize clinicians to the clinical scenarios which could lead to confusion in diagnosis with subsequent delay in management.

I hope this book will benefit clinicians in managing patients with invasive fungal rhinosinusitis.

Acknowledgements

This book saw the light of day due to my patients of invasive fungal sinusitis who have taught me so much; Dr. Kirtane, my teacher, who has provided me tremendous encouragement; my husband, Dinesh Vartak, and mom for their support; my contributors (Dr. Soman, Dr. Anjali Shetty, Dr. Santosh Gupta and Dr. Maheshwari) who kept to the deadline despite their busy schedules; Dr. Camilla Rodrigues, who reviewed the draft for factual errors; Mr. Pramod Tandel, photographer, who helped improve the resolutions of the pictures; the management and trustees of P.D. Hinduja Hospital for providing the atmosphere for academics despite being a busy corporate hospital; and finally my publishers, Springer-Verlag, especially Dr. Naren Aggarwal and Dr. Eti Dinesh who provided help, advice and encouragement. I thank you all.

Contents

Introduction

Gauri Mankekar

Invasive fungal sinusitis is defined as the presence of fungal hyphae within the mucosa, submucosa, bone, or blood vessels on histopathology [1]. Once considered a rare disorder, today it is being reported with increasing frequency around the world. Invasive zygomycosis followed by invasive aspergillosis is an important concern in India as the world's highest number of cases of zygomycosis are being reported from here [2]. It is often misdiagnosed or there is a delay in diagnosis resulting in high rate of morbidity as well as mortality. Successful patient outcome depends on high index of clinical suspicion; adequate and appropriate sinus biopsies; rapid microbiological, pathological, and radiological diagnosis; followed by prompt aggressive and concomitant surgical debridement, antifungal treatment, and management of the underlying or predisposing metabolic or other systemic disorders.

Of the approximately 1.5 billion [3] fungal species supposedly existing in the world, approximately 400 are human pathogens, and again, only 50 of these cause systemic or central nervous system infections. Many of these are ubiquitous in our environment. Although many humans are colonized by fungi, an intact immune system prevents subsequent infection [4] as well as its progression.

Invasive fungal sinusitis is usually seen in immunocompromised individuals. Factors predisposing to the development of invasive fungal sinusitis include [1, 2, 5–8]:

- Metabolic or systemic disorders

  - Diabetes mellitus
  - Hematological disorders, e.g., leukemia, lymphomas, and aplastic anemia
  - Hemochromatosis
  - Acquired immunodeficiency syndrome (AIDS)

G. Mankekar, MS, DNB, PhD
ENT, PD Hinduja Hospital, Mahim, Mumbai,
Maharashtra 400 016, India
e-mail: gaurimankekar@gmail.com

G. Mankekar (ed.), *Invasive Fungal Rhinosinusitis,*
DOI 10.1007/978-81-322-1530-1_1, © Springer India 2014

- Iatrogenic immunosuppression
  - Systemic steroid therapy
  - Chemotherapy with neutropenia
  - Prolonged antibiotic therapy
- Post-organ or stem cell transplantation

Occasionally invasive fungal sinusitis may occur in immunocompetent individuals [1, 7, 8]. Noninvasive fungal disease may progress to invasive disease (mixed infection) if the immunological status of a patient changes. Such a progression may be precipitated by a change of host defenses [9], and the diagnosis of "invasion of tissue" in such cases requires an experienced histopathologist.

The best outcome reported in acute fulminant invasive fungal sinusitis is near 50 % survival [1]. To improve survival rates, clinicians must be aware of the manifestations of the disease and have access to good diagnostic mycology and pathology laboratories for rapid diagnosis which is essential for the management of this disease. Only a multidisciplinary management approach can ensure successful outcomes in patients of invasive fungal sinusitis.

References

1. de Shazo RD, O'Brien M, Chapin K, et al. A new classification and diagnostic criteria for invasive fungal sinusitis. Arch Otolaryngol Head Neck Surg. 1997;123(11):1181–8.
2. Chakrabarti A, Chatterjee SS, Shivaprakash MR. Overview of opportunistic fungal infections in India. J Med Mycol. 2008;49:165–72.
3. Hawksworth DL. The magnitude of fungal diversity: the 1.5 million species estimate revisited. Mycol Res. 2001;105:1422–32.
4. Bazan 3rd C, Rinaldi MG, Rauch RR, Jinkins JR. Fungal infections of the brain. Neuroimaging Clin N Am. 1991;1:57–88.
5. Epstein VA, Kern RC. Invasive fungal sinusitis and complications of rhinosinusitis. Otolaryngol Clin North Am. 2008;41:497–524.
6. Stringer SP, Ryan MW. Chronic invasive fungal rhinosinusitis. Otolaryngol Clin North Am. 2000;33(2):375–87.
7. Gillespie MB, O'Malley BW. An algorithmic approach to the diagnosis and management of invasive fungal rhinosinusitis in the immunocompromised patient. Otolaryngol Clin North Am. 2000;33(2):323–34.
8. Sridhara SR, Paragache G, Panda NK, et al. Mucormycosis in immunocompetent individuals: an increasing trend. J Otolaryngol. 2005;34(6):402–6.
9. Gungor A, Adusumilli V, Corey JP. Fungal sinusitis progression of disease in immunosuppression – a case report. Ear Nose Throat J. 1998;77:207–15.

Classification of Fungal Sinusitis

Gauri Mankekar

The classification of fungal sinusitis has gradually evolved over the past several decades. Classification is essential to choose appropriate management strategies as well as to predict prognosis. The first distinction between invasive and noninvasive sinusitis was made by Hora [1] in 1965 on the basis of clinical findings. Chronic granulomatous sinusitis was first described in Sudan in 1967, and subsequent cases were reported from Pakistan, India, and also from the USA [2–4]. In 1976, Safirstein [5] reported a combination of nasal polyposis, crusting, and Aspergillus species in sinus cultures similar to those seen in allergic bronchopulmonary aspergillosis (ABPA). In 1980, McGill [6] et al. reported a fulminant form of fungal rhinosinusitis with a malignant course in immunocompromised patients. Also, in 1980, Talbot et al. [7] presented a classification of invasive fungal sinusitis as (1) fulminant aspergillosis, (2) rhinocerebral mucormycosis, and (3) aspergilloma. In 1988, invasive sinusitis was classified as acute invasive and chronic invasive in a review of chronic sinusitis in normal hosts [4]. Meanwhile, several clinicians, individually [8–12] recognized cases of chronic rhinosinusitis associated with a mucosal plug in sinuses of patients with ABPA, and this led to the renaming of this type of fungal rhinosinusitis as allergic fungal sinusitis or rhinosinusitis (AFS or AFRS). Ponikau et al. [13] have proposed the term "eosinophilic fungal rhinosinusitis" to reflect the important feature "eosinophils."

In 1997, DeShazo et al. [14], proposed diagnostic criteria and classification for invasive fungal sinusitis and in subsequent publications [15, 16], proposed two types of non-invasive fungal sinusitis: allergic fungal sinusitis and sinus mycetoma or fungal ball and three types of invasive fungal sinusitis:

1. Acute fulminant
2. Chronic invasive
3. Chronic granulomatous invasive

G. Mankekar, MS, DNB, PhD
ENT, PD Hinduja Hospital, Mahim, Mumbai,
Maharashtra 400 016, India
e-mail: gaurimankekar@gmail.com

G. Mankekar (ed.), *Invasive Fungal Rhinosinusitis*,
DOI 10.1007/978-81-322-1530-1_2, © Springer India 2014

The diagnostic criterion for invasive fungal sinusitis was based on histopathological evidence of hyphal forms within the sinus mucosa, submucosa, blood vessels, or bone. On the other hand, in mucosa of patients with chronic bacterial sinusitis or in patients of allergic fungal sinusitis and mycetoma, there is absence of stainable hyphae [16].

Invasive fungal sinusitis is defined as acute when the duration is less than 4 weeks, while disease of more than 4 weeks duration is said to be chronic [17].

Acute Fulminant Invasive Fungal Sinusitis

Acute fulminant invasive fungal sinusitis is a rapidly progressing invasive disease usually seen in immunocompromised patients [16]. The disease can have a rapid downhill course over few days to weeks. Rapid spread of the infection occurs as a result of vascular invasion by the fungus, leading to vascular thrombosis and tissue infarction.

Chronic Invasive Fungal Sinusitis

Chronic invasive fungal sinusitis is a relatively rare type of invasive fungal sinusitis seen usually in diabetic or immunocompetent patients with disease progression occurring over more than 12 weeks [16].

Granulomatous Invasive Fungal Sinusitis

Granulomatous invasive fungal sinusitis also has an indolent course and is usually seen in immunocompetent individuals with patients usually presenting with proptosis. This type of fungal sinusitis has been reported from Sudan, India, and Pakistan [2–4, 16].

The American Academy of Otolaryngology Head and Neck Surgery and other related societies attempted a consensus of definition, classification, and suggested clinical strategies for patients with rhinosinusitis [18].

They divided rhinosinusitis into four categories: acute (bacterial) rhinosinusitis, chronic rhinosinusitis (CRS) without polyps, CRS with polyps, and allergic fungal sinusitis. The spectrum of fungal involvement in CRS was considered from benign colonization to potentially life-threatening invasive disease.

A consensus panel discussed this classification addressing the controversies in 2009 [19]. They recommended that based on histopathological evidence of tissue invasion by fungi, fungal rhinosinusitis be classified as (Fig. 1) invasive and noninvasive diseases. The invasive diseases include (1) acute invasive (fulminant) FRS, (2) chronic invasive FRS, and (3) granulomatous invasive FRS. The noninvasive

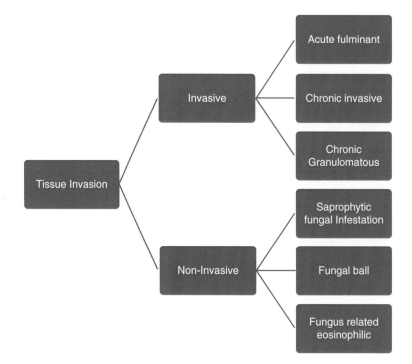

Fig. 1 Classification of fungal sinusitis based on tissue invasion. After Chakrabarti et al. [19]

diseases include (1) saprophytic fungal infestation, (2) fungal ball, and (3) fungus-related eosinophilic FRS that includes AFRS.

Saprophytic fungal infestation: This is described as asymptomatic colonization of mucous crusts within the sino-nasal cavity, often in patients who have undergone previous sinus surgery. It has been predicted that this growth could lead to the formation of fungal ball [17].

Fungal ball: It is described as accumulation of dense conglomeration of fungal hyphae, without invasion, in one sinus cavity, usually the maxillary sinus, although the disease may affect other sinuses or rarely multiple sinuses [20]. It has been designated by various terms such as mycetoma, aspergilloma, and chronic non-invasive granuloma [17].

Fungus-related eosinophilic FRS that includes AFRS: The Bent and Kuhn [12] diagnostic criteria to diagnose AFRS are type I hypersensitivity, nasal polyposis, characteristic CT findings, presence of fungi on direct microscopy or culture, and allergic mucin containing fungal elements without tissue invasion. It is believed that eosinophilic rhinosinusitis (EMRS) and AFRS are differing manifestations of the same pathological process, with considerable overlap [19].

Irrespective of the controversy regarding classification of fungal sinusitis, it is extremely important to investigate all patients of chronic rhinosinusitis not responding to standard therapy and to identify the invasive versus the noninvasive form (allergic fungal sinusitis, fungal mycetoma). Aggressive surgery and antifungal treatment is required in the invasive forms while surgery alone may suffice in the non-invasive forms [21].

References

1. Hora JF. Primary aspergillosis of the paranasal sinuses and associated areas. Laryngoscope. 1965;75:768–73.
2. Chakrabarti A, Sharma SC, Chander J. Epidemiology and pathogenesis of paranasal sinus mycoses. Otolaryngol Head Neck Surg. 1992;107:745–50.
3. Hussain S, Salahuddin N, Ahmad I, Jooma R. Rhinocerebral invasive mycosis: occurrence in immunocompetent individuals. Eur J Radiol. 1995;20:151–5.
4. Washburn RG, Kennedy DW, Begley MG, Henderson DK, Bennett JE. Chronic fungal sinusitis in apparently normal hosts. Medicine. 1988;67:231–47.
5. Safirstein B. Allergic bronchopulmonary aspergillosis with obstruction of the upper respiratory tract. Chest. 1976;70:788–90.
6. McGill TJ, Simpson G, Healy GB. Fulminant aspergillosis of the nose and paranasal sinuses: a new clinical entity. Laryngoscope. 1980;90:748–54.
7. Talbot GH, Huang A, Provencher M. Invasive aspergillus rhinosinusitis in patients with acute leukemia. Rev Infect Dis. 1991;13:219–32.
8. Millar JN, Johnston A, Lamb D. Allergic aspergillosis of the maxillary sinuses. Thorax. 1981; 36:710.
9. Katzenstein AA, Sole SR, Greenberger PA. Allergic aspergillus sinusitis: a newly recognized form of sinusitis. J Allergy Clin Immunol. 1983;72:82–93.
10. Allphin AL, Strauss M, Abdul Karim FW. Allergic fungal sinusitis: problems in diagnosis and treatment. Laryngoscope. 1991;101:815–20.
11. Manning SC, Schaefer SD, Close LG, Vuitch F. Culture positive allergic fungal sinusitis. Arch Otolaryngol. 1991;117:174–8.
12. Bent JP, Kuhn FA. Diagnosis of allergic fungal sinusitis. Otolaryngol Head Neck Surg. 1994; 111:580–8.
13. Ponikau JU, Sherris DA, Kern EB, et al. The diagnosis and incidence of allergic fungal sinusitis. Mayo Clin Proc. 1999;74:877–84.
14. deShazo RD, O'Brien M, Chapin K, Sato-Aguilar M, Gardner L, Swain RE. A new classification and diagnostic criteria for invasive fungal sinusitis. Arch Otolaryngol Head Neck Surgery. 1997;123:1181–8.
15. deShazo RD, Swain RE. Diagnostic criteria for allergic fungal sinusitis. J Allergy Clin Immunol. 1995;96:24–35.
16. deShazo RD, O'Brien M, Chapin K. Criteria for the diagnosis of sinus mycetoma. J Allergy Clin Immunol. 1997;99:475–85.
17. Ferguson BJ. Definitions of fungal rhinosinusitis. Otolaryngol Clin North Am. 2000; 33(2):227–35.
18. Meltzer E, Hamilos D, Hadley J, et al. Rhinosinusitis: establishing definitions for clinical research and patient care. J Allergy Clin Immunol. 2004;114(Suppl):S155–22.
19. Chakrabarti A, Denning DW, Ferguson B, et al. Fungal rhinosinusitis: a categorization and definitional schema addressing current controversies. Laryngoscope. 2009;119(9):1809–18.
20. Grosjean P, Weber R. Fungus balls of the paranasal sinuses: a review. Eur Arch Otorhinolaryngol. 2007;264:461–70.
21. Chakrabarti A, Das A, Panda NK. Overview of fungal sinusitis- guest editorial. Indian J Otolaryngol Head Neck Surg. 2004;56(4):251–8.

Epidemiology, Pathogenesis, and Risk Factors

Gauri Mankekar

Invasive fungal sinusitis has been reported from all over the world, but its incidence varies widely with higher frequency reported in Sudan [1], southwestern states of the USA, and India, which have a hot and dry climate. The incidence seems to be higher in India than elsewhere in the world [2]. The true incidence of mucormycosis is unknown and probably underestimated due to the difficulties in antemortem diagnosis and the low autopsy rates in patients who die in the setting of either leukemia or stem cell transplant [3]. However, there is a consensus that there has been an overall increase in the incidence of all types of fungal sinusitis [2, 4]. At M.D. Anderson Cancer Center, Texas, the number of reported cases increased from 8 per 100,000 admissions during 1989–1993 to 17 per 100,000 admissions during 1994–1998 [4].

Seasonal variation in the incidence of Mucorales infection has been suggested by some authors. Talmi et al. [5], from Israel, noted that 16 of their 19 cases of rhino-orbito-cerebral mucormycosis occurred between August and November, while Funada et al., from Japan, reported six of seven cases having developed between August and September [6].

Many environmental and host factors have been postulated to contribute to the development of fungal sinusitis. Inhaled fungal spores seem to be converted from saprophytic to pathogenic fungi in the presence of sinus obstruction with impairment of the sinus ventilation [2]. As higher incidence of fungal sinusitis is reported from regions with warm and dry climate, it has been postulated that dusty, arid conditions predispose to rhinitis and recurrent sinusitis, facilitating the growth of saprophytic fungi [2]. It is believed that hot, dry, and dusty climate produces inflammation and mucositis, allowing an ingrowth and tissue damage by the fungus and its metabolites. This is followed by both an immediate and delayed hypersensitivity

G. Mankekar, MS, DNB, PhD
ENT, PD Hinduja Hospital, Mahim, Mumbai,
Maharashtra 400 016, India
e-mail: gaurimankekar@gmail.com

G. Mankekar (ed.), *Invasive Fungal Rhinosinusitis*,
DOI 10.1007/978-81-322-1530-1_3, © Springer India 2014

reaction of the host to the fungal antigens, leading to fungal sinusitis [7]. Another probability to be considered is of rhinosinusitis treated with antibiotics and local intranasal steroids altering the paranasal sinus flora, the local mucosal immunity, and pH of the sinus mucosa and secretions providing an environment for inhaled fungal spores to become pathogenic especially in diabetics and immunocompromised individuals.

Several host factors are known to predispose to invasive fungal sinusitis, and the fulminant form is common in immunocompromised hosts [1–7]. It has been reported in patients with diabetes, especially with ketoacidosis [8], hematological conditions (neutropenia {with counts less than 500 neutrophils/mm^4}, leukemia, lymphoma, multiple myeloma, myelodysplastic syndrome, aplastic anemia, and sideroblastic anemia) [9–11], HIV [12], cirrhosis, carcinoma, hepatitis, glomerulonephritis, uremia [13], bone marrow [14] and stem cell transplantation [15], solid organ transplantation [16, 17], and immunosuppressive therapy (steroids or chemotherapy) received in the month before diagnosis [4]. Invasive fungal sinusitis affects approximately 0.9–1.9 % of allogenic bone marrow transplant recipients [14].

Patients with solid tumors rarely develop invasive fungal infections. Kontoyiannis et al. [4] did not find any cases of invasive fungal infections among patients with solid tumors over a 10-year period.

Hematological malignancy is a major risk factor for invasive fungal sinusitis, especially mucormycosis, with leukemia or lymphoma being the underlying diagnosis in the majority of patients [19]. Forty to hundred percent of patients with hematological conditions were neutropenic at diagnosis [4, 14]. The median duration of neutropenia before diagnosis was reported to be 16 days [4]. In patients with hematological conditions, pulmonary, followed by disseminated and rhino-orbito-cerebral mucormycosis are most common [4], while in patients with diabetes, especially with ketoacidosis, rhino-orbito-cerebral mucormycosis is most common [20].

Patients with solid organ transplants are particularly at risk for invasive fungal infections, especially if they have been treated with high-dose steroids, OKT3, or anti-thymocyte globulin [16, 17]. Liver transplant recipients are at high risk for invasive fungal infections due to the high intraoperative blood transfusion requirement (causing iron overload), bacterial infections, and re-transplantation for graft failure [17].

Desferroxamine therapy for iron or aluminum overload, especially in patients requiring hemodialysis is associated with mucormycosis [21, 22]. Patients with other iron overload conditions requiring desferroxamine therapy such as myelodysplastic syndrome, beta-thalassemia, and sideroblastic anemia are also known to have developed mucormycosis [22]. Daly et al. [22] found that one-half of the patients had disseminated infection while one-quarter had isolated rhinocerebral disease. They also observed a mortality rate of 90 % in these patients. Desferroxamine acts as a siderophore to promote the growth of mucormycosis

[26, 27]. Today, fewer cases of mucormycosis are expected in dialysis patients since therapeutic erythropoietin has reduced the need for frequent blood transfusions [8].

Iron overload, on its own, is also known to be a risk factor for invasive fungal infections [11, 15, 23]. Iron overload is common in MDS, beta-thalassemia and sideroblastic anemia, and in patients receiving excessive blood transfusions intraoperatively during liver transplantation. Iron overload has also been associated with the risk of invasive fungal infections after allogeneic hematopoietic stem cell transplant (HCT) [15]. It is believed that iron overload may increase the risk of infection through at least two mechanisms: First, this may be a direct effect of free iron on bacterial and fungal growth [24, 35]. Iron is a necessary growth factor for many microorganisms [25]. In animal models of mucormycosis, iron and desferroxamine promote growth and increase the virulence of *Rhizopus oryzae* and *Rhizopus microsporus* [26, 27]. Secondly, excess free iron impairs the natural resistance to infection, through complex mechanisms including inhibition of IFN-gamma, TNF-alpha, IL-12, nitric oxide formation, and impairment of macrophage, neutrophil, and T-cell functions [28, 29].

Diabetics, especially those with ketoacidosis, are more at risk of rhino-orbito-cerebral mucormycosis [8]. Normal serum inhibits the growth of Mucorales [26]. In vitro, serum acidosis permits growth of *Rhizopus* spp. [26]. Artis et al. [30] and Boelaert et al. [26] have shown that acidosis inhibits transferrin's capacity to bind iron, thus allowing *Rhizopus* spp. to use it for growth in vitro. Artis et al. [30] found that serum of four of seven diabetic patients with ketoacidosis incubated with *R. oryzae* spores supported profuse growth but inhibited growth when pH was titrated to 7.4. The three samples which did not support growth had significantly lower iron levels. Also serum glucose level did not influence growth irrespective of pH [30]. In diabetics, impaired neutrophil and macrophage function may also contribute to an increased risk of mucormycosis [31].

When rhino-orbito-cerebral mucormycosis develops in an immunocompetent host, *Apophysomyces elegans* should be considered as a likely pathogen [32].

Another emerging risk factor for zygomycosis is long-term therapy with voriconazole as prophylaxis for treatment of invasive fungal infections in hematopoietic stem cell transplantation or patients with hematologic malignancies [18]. Breakthrough mucormycosis is increasingly being observed in these patients receiving Aspergillus-active drugs such as voriconazole or the echinocandins, as both these agents have no anti-Mucorales activity [33].

In view of the multiple, interrelated risk factors (Fig. 1) present in most patients of invasive fungal infections, it is often impossible to ascribe a single risk factor that increases the risk or worsens the prognosis of this devastating infection [34].

Documented mucormycosis is at least five to ten times less common as compared to other mold infections such as Aspergillosis, making it difficult for

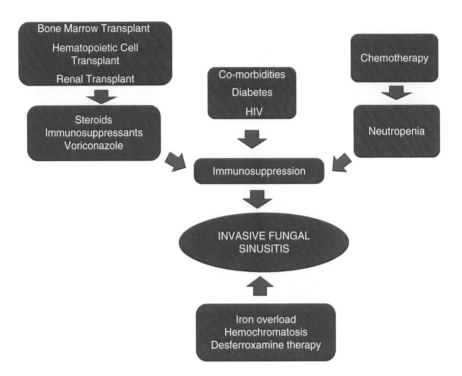

Fig. 1 Risk factors for invasive fungal sinusitis – many of them are interrelated

inexperienced personnel to identify the infection early [3]. As the pathophysiology, mode of acquisition, and underlying patient risk factors for mucormycosis are similar to aspergillosis, clinical distinction between the two entities is difficult [36]. Both infections are acquired primarily through inhalation of fungal spores, which are ubiquitous in the environment, leading to sinopulmonary disease [37–39] (Fig. 2). However, some scenarios, risk factors, and elements of clinical and radiological features could prompt to a high index of suspicion for incipient mucormycosis [18, 35] (Table 1).

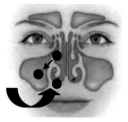

Inhaled fungal spores trapped in the paranasal sinuses

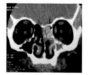

Macrophages and PMN block replication (impaired in neutropenic patients or with corticosteroid, moAb therapy of graft vs host disease or hyperglycemia)

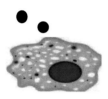

undetected fungal proliferation, angioinvasion, necrosis. (fungal proliferation enhanced with iron overload)

Progressing fungal invasion, hemorrhage and necrosis detectable by CT scan

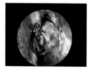

extensive necrosis limits drug delivery and immune response

Dissemination

Fig. 2 Pathophysiology of invasive fungal sinusitis (Based on Pathophysiology of invasive pulmonary mucormycosis: Kontoyiannis and Lewis [36])

Table 1 Factors favoring mucormycosis over aspergillosis (Kontoyiannis and Lewis [36])

Clues	Comments
Epidemiology and host clues	
Institution with high rates of mucormycosis	Unique geographic exposures vs. institution-specific differences in immunosuppression and anti-infective practices
Iron overload	Most reliable method of diagnosis unclear
Hyperglycemia with or without diabetes mellitus	Degree and duration undefined
Prior voriconazole or echinocandin use	The magnitude and specificity of such association are debatable
Clinical, radiologic, and laboratory clues	
Community-acquired sinusitis	Pansinusitis or ethmoid involvement are important clinical clues of mucormycosis
Oral or necrotic lesions on hard palate or turbinates	
Chest wall cellulitis adjacent to lung infarct	Mucormycosis can spread across tissue planes
Acute vascular event (e.g., myocardial infarct, GI bleeding)	Resulting from acute hemorrhagic infarct caused by Mucorales
Reverse halo sign on CXR or CT	Halo sign is as common in invasive pulmonary mucor as in invasive pulmonary aspergillosis
Presumed (by CT findings) fungal pneumonia with adequate voriconazole levels	
Presumed (by CT findings) fungal pneumonia with repetitively negative galactomannan and G-glucan serum levels	

References

1. Veress B, Malik OA, Tayeb AA, El Daoud S, El Mahgoub S, El Hassan AM. Further observations on the primary paranasal Aspergillus granuloma in Sudan. Am J Trop Med Hyg. 1973;22:765–72.
2. Chakrabarti A, Sharma SC. Paranasal sinus mycoses. Indian J Chest Dis Allied Sci. 2000; 42:293–304.
3. Chamilos G, Luna M, Lewis RE, et al. Invasive fungal infections in patients with hematologic malignancies in a tertiary care cancer center: an autopsy study over a 15 year period (1989–2003). Haematologica. 2006;91(7):986–9.
4. Kontoyiannis DP, Wessel VC, Bodey GP, Rolston VI. Zygomycosis in the 1990s in a tertiary care cancer center. Clin Infect Dis. 2000;30:851–6.
5. Talmi YP, Goldschmeid-Reouven A, Bakon M, et al. Rhino-orbital and rhino-orbito-cerebral mucormycosis. Otolaryngol Head Neck Surg. 2002;127:22–31.
6. Funada H, Matsuda T. Pulmonary mucormycosis in a hematology ward. Intern Med. 1996;35:540–4.
7. Chakrabarti A, Sharma SC, Chander J. Epidemiology and pathogenesis of paranasal sinus mycoses. Otolaryngol Head Neck Surg. 1992;107:745–50.
8. Prabhu RM, Patel R. Mucormycosis and entomophthoramycosis: a review of the clinical manifestations, diagnosis and treatment. Clin Microbiol Infect. 2004;10 Suppl 1:31–47.
9. Herbrecht R, Letscher-Bru V, Bowden RA, et al. Treatment of 21 cases of invasive mucormycosis with amphotericin B colloidal dispersion. Eur J Clin Microbiol Infect Dis. 2001;20: 460–6.

10. Mileshkin L, Slavin M, Seymour JF, McKenzie A. Successful treatment of rhinocerebral zygomycosis using liposomal nystatin. Leuk Lymphoma. 2001;42:1119–23.
11. Wueppenhorst N, Lee M-K, Rappold E, Kayser G, Beckervordersandforth J, de With K, Serr A. Rhino-orbitocerebral zygomycosis caused by Conidiobolus incongruous in an immunocompromised patient in Germany. J Clin Microbiol. 2010;48(11):4322–5. doi: 10.1128/JCM.01188-10. Epub 2010 Sep 22.
12. Hejny C, Kerrison JB, Newman NJ, Stone CM. Rhino-orbital mucormycosis in a patient with acquired immunodeficiency syndrome (AIDS) and neutropenia. Am J Ophthalmol. 2001;132: 111–2.
13. Lehrer RI, Howard DH, et al. Mucormycosis. Ann Intern Med. 1980;9:93–108.
14. Baddley JW, Stroud TP, Salzman D, Pappas PG. Invasive mold infections in allogenic bone transplant recipients. Clin Infect Dis. 2001;32:1319–24.
15. Kontoyiannis DP, Chamilos G, Lewis RE, et al. Increased bone marrow iron stores is an independent risk factor for invasive aspergillosis in patients with high risk hematologic malignancies and recipients of allogenic hematopoietic stem cell transplantation. Cancer. 2007;110(6): 1303–6.
16. Morduchowicz G, Shmueli D, Shapira Z, et al. Rhinocerebral mucormycosis in renal transplant recipients: report of three cases and review of literature. Rev Infect Dis. 1986;8: 441–6.
17. Jimenez C, Lumbreras C, Paseiro G, et al. Treatment of mucor infection after liver or pancreas-kidney transplantation. Transplant Proc. 2002;34:82–3.
18. Trifilio SM, et al. Breakthrough zygomycosis after voriconazole administration among patients with hematologic malignancies who receive hematopoietic stem-cell transplants or intensive chemotherapy. Bone Marrow Transplant. 2007;39:425.
19. Ingram CW, Sennesh J, Cooper JN, Perfect JR. Disseminated zygomycosis. Report of four cases and review. Rev Infect Dis. 1989;11:741–54.
20. Espinel-Ingroff A, Oakley LA, Kerkering TM. Opportunistic zygomycotic infections. Mycopathologica. 1987;97:33–41.
21. Boelaert JR, Fenves AZ, Coburn JW. Mucormycosis among patients on dialysis. N Engl J Med. 1989;321:190–1.
22. Daly AL, Velazquez LA, Bradley SF, Kauffman CA. Mucormycosis: association with deferoxamine therapy. Am J Med. 1989;87:468–71.
23. Toma A, Fenaux P, Dreyfus F, Cordonnier C. Infections in myelodysplastic syndromes. Haematologica. 2012;97(10):1459–70.
24. Lounis N, Truffot-Pernot C, Grosset J, Gordeuk VR, Boelaert JR. Iron and mycobacterium tuberculosis infection. J Clin Virol. 2001;20(3):123–6.
25. Schaible UE, Kauffman SH. Iron and microbial infection. Nat Rev Microbiol. 2004;2(12): 946–53.
26. Boelaert JR, Locht M, Van Cutsem J, et al. Mucormycosis during deferoxamine therapy is a siderophore mediated infection. In vitro and in vivo animal studies. J Clin Invest. 1993;91: 1979–86.
27. Abe F, Inaba H, Katoh T, Hotchi M. Effects of iron and deferoxamine on Rhizopus infection. Mycopathologica. 1990;110:87–90.
28. Bullen JJ, Rogers HJ, Spalding PB, Ward CG. Natural resistance, iron and infection: a challenge for clinical medicine. J Med Microbiol. 2006;55(3):251–8.
29. Boelaert JR Vandecasteele SJ, Appelberg R, Gordeuk VR. The effect of the host's iron status on tuberculosis. J Infect Dis. 2007;195(12):1745–53.
30. Artis WM, Fountain JA, Delcher HK, Jones HE. A mechanism of susceptibility to mucormycosis in diabetic ketoacidosis: transferrin and iron availability. Mycopathologica. 1990;110: 87–90.
31. Mowat AG, Baum J. Chemotaxis of polymorphonuclear leukocytes from patients with diabetes mellitus. N Engl J Med. 1971;284:621–7.

32. Garcia-Covarrubias L, Bartlett R, Bartlett DM, Wasserman RJ. Rhino-orbito-cerebral mucormycosis attributed to Apophysomyces elegans in an immunocompetent individual: a case report and review of literature. J Trauma. 2001;50:353–7.
33. Boucher HW, Groll AH, Chiou CC, Walsh TJ. Newer systemic antifungal agents: pharmacokinetics, safety and efficacy. Drugs. 2004;64(18):1997–2020.
34. Pongas GN, Lewis RE, Samonis G, Kontoyiannis DP. Voriconazole associated zygomycosis: a significant consequence of evolving antifungal prophylaxis and immunosuppression practices? Clin Microbiol Infect. 2009;15(50):93–7.
35. Kontoyiannis DP, Lionakis MS, Lewis RE, et al. Zygomycosis in a tertiary care cancer center in the era of Aspergillus active anti fungal therapy: a case controlled observational study of 27 recent cases. J Infect Dis. 2005;191(8):1350–60.
36. Kontoyiannis DP, Lewis RE. How I treat mucormycosis. Blood. 2011;118(5):1216–24.
37. Spellberg B, Edwards Jr J, Ibrahim A. Novel perspectives on mucormycosis: pathophysiology, presentation and management. Clin Microbiol Rev. 2005;18(3):556–69.
38. Roden MM, Zaoutis TE, Buchanan WL, et al. Epidemiology and outcome of zygomycosis: a review of 929 reported cases. Clin Infect Dis. 2005;41(5):634–53.
39. Kontoyiannis DP, Lewis RE. Invasive zygomycosis: an update on pathogenesis, clinical manifestations and management. Infect Dis Clin North Am. 2006;20(3):581–607.

Clinical Features and Diagnosis

Gauri Mankekar and Kashmira Chavan

Invasive fungal sinusitis can be diagnosed early only if the primary clinician treating the patient, whether an ENT surgeon, a chemotherapist, an oncologist or a paediatrician, has a high index of clinical suspicion. In addition, there should be both microbiological as well as histopathological evidence for further definitive management. An analysis of tissue invasion and host immunological response is an important step in the evaluation of the patient.

The clinical features of the disease vary depending upon the acuity of the fungal infection. While acute invasive fungal sinusitis is a rapidly progressing infection, chronic invasive and granulomatous are indolent and progress insidiously over several months to years.

Acute Invasive Fungal Sinusitis

It is the most lethal form of fungal sinusitis, and the incidence of reported mortality is 50–80 % [1]. It is usually seen in immunocompromised individuals but is also seen occasionally in immunocompetent persons. It is also postulated that the nasal cavity is the primary site of infection, with the middle turbinate being affected in two-thirds of the biopsy positive cases [2].

Initially patient may complain of nasal block with bloodstained or serosanguineous nasal discharge. There may be painless, necrotic nasal septal ulcer or eschar.

G. Mankekar, MS, DNB, PhD (✉)
ENT, PD Hinduja Hospital, Mahim, Mumbai,
Maharashtra 400 016, India
e-mail: gaurimankekar@gmail.com

K. Chavan, DNB (ENT)
Department of ENT, Former Clinical Associate, Khar Hinduja Healthcare, Khar, Mumbai,
Maharashtra, India

G. Mankekar (ed.), *Invasive Fungal Rhinosinusitis*,
DOI 10.1007/978-81-322-1530-1_4, © Springer India 2014

Fig. 1 Stage 1: Early
rhino-maxillary fungal
sinusitis

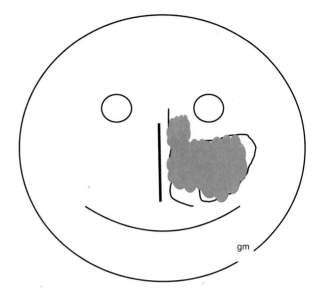

There is rapid progression over a few days with angioinvasion and haematogenous dissemination with fungi invading the mucosa, submucosa, blood vessels and bony walls of the nose and paranasal sinuses. Hyperglycemia and acidosis provide ideal conditions for fungal growth and tissue invasion. Also ketoacidosis has been shown to adversely affect phagocytic activity [3]. There may be intracranial spread either through the cribriform plate or via the orbital apex or via septic emboli. Once the ophthalmic and other orbital arteries are involved, infection can further reach the cavernous sinus and carotid artery. Acute subdural hematoma, cavernous sinus thrombosis and internal carotid artery thrombosis may occur in rhinocerebral mucormycosis. Invasion of the carotid arteries can rapidly lead to cerebral ischemia and death [4, 5].

Depending upon the progression of the infection, Spellberg et al. [6] classified it as:

Stage 1: Rhinomaxillary (Fig. 1; Figs. 1, 2, 3 in Chapter "Radiology in Invasive Fungal Sinusitis")
Stage 2: Rhino-orbital (Fig 2; Figs. 4, 5, 6 in Chapter "Radiology in Invasive Fungal Sinusitis")
Stage 3: Rhino-orbito-cerebral (Fig. 3; Fig. 7 in Chapter "Radiology in Invasive Fungal Sinusitis")

Symptoms

The following symptoms, especially in an immunocompromised patient, should arouse the suspicion of fungal disease:

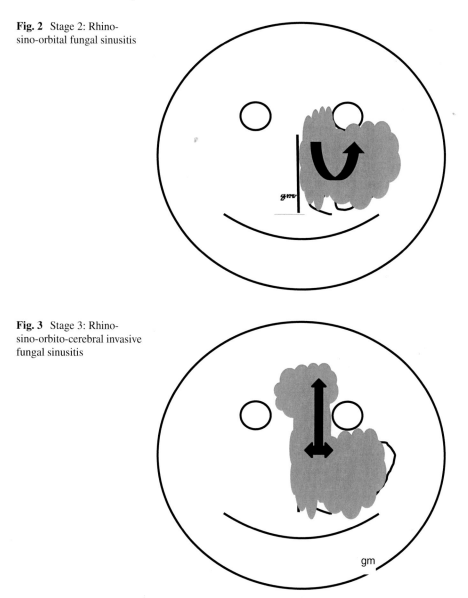

Fig. 2 Stage 2: Rhino-sino-orbital fungal sinusitis

Fig. 3 Stage 3: Rhino-sino-orbito-cerebral invasive fungal sinusitis

- Fever with spikes, not responding to antibiotics. It is the most common presenting feature [7].
- Persistent nasal blockage with bloodstained serosanguineous nasal discharge with cough.
- With progression of the disease, there could be facial or periorbital swelling (Fig. 4), facial pain, numbness and headache.
- Orbital symptoms: Spread of disease to orbit may cause chemosis, proptosis, ptosis, blurring of vision, loss of vision and ophthalmoplegia.

Fig. 4 Facial and periorbital
(*arrow*) swelling

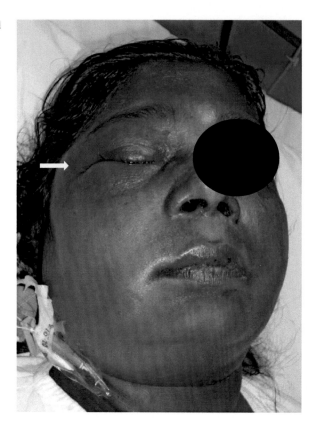

- Cranial nerve palsies especially 2nd, 3rd, 4th, 5th, 6th and 7th nerve due to cavernous sinus thrombosis or temporal lobe mycotic infarcts.
- CNS symptoms such as altered consciousness, delirium, convulsions, hemiparesis, hemiplegia or coma may be seen in patients with intracranial involvement.

Examination

The patient is usually under treatment with a physician for a metabolic disorder or oncologist for chemotherapy with neutropenia and then referred to either an ENT surgeon or an ophthalmologist.

ENT Examination

Initial or a cursory nasal examination may not reveal anything significant. Therefore, it is always advisable to decongest the nose and perform nasal endoscopy. A discolouration of the nasal mucosa and serosanguineous discharge should

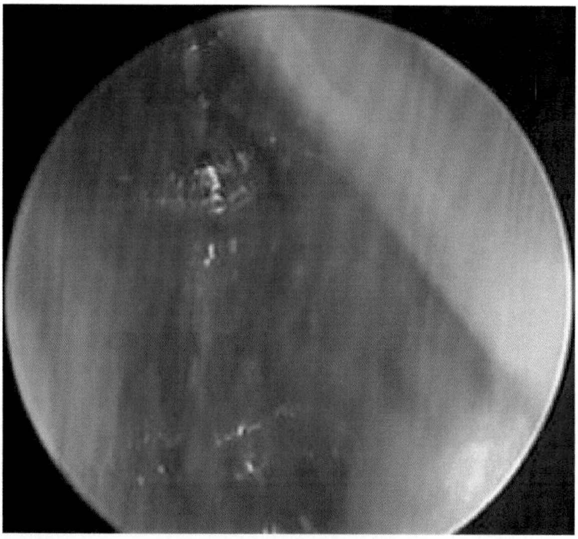

Fig. 5 Endoscopic appearance of discoloured nasal mucosa in a case of mucormycosis

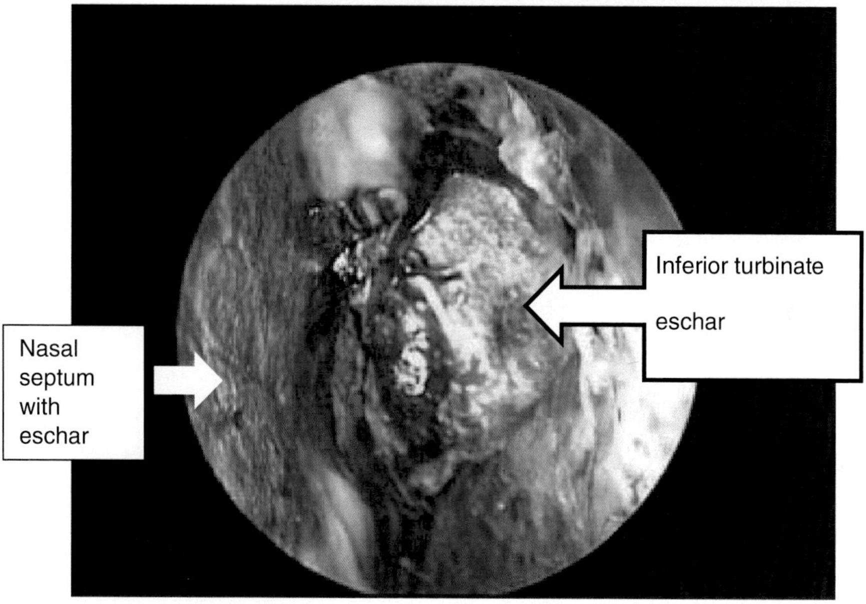

Inferior turbinate eschar

Nasal septum with eschar

Fig. 6 Progressive nasal septal and lateral nasal wall infarction (*arrows*) in a case of acute fulminant mucormycosis

be looked for. Crusting, whitish discolouration (due to tissue ischemia) (Fig. 5) or black discolouration with eschar formation (Fig. 6) (due to tissue necrosis) may be present [8]. There could also be granulation or ulceration of the nasal mucosa. These changes have been most commonly found to occur on the middle turbinate, followed by the septum, palate and inferior turbinate [9]. There may be reduced

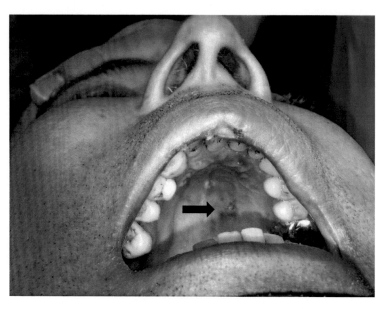

Fig. 7 Discolouration of palate (*black arrow*) in early palatal involvement in a diabetic patient with rhino-orbital mucormycosis

Fig. 8 Palatal infarction (*white arrow*) in progressive mucormycosis

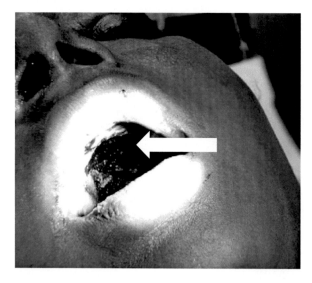

nasal mucosal bleeding on account of tissue ischemia or infarction. The sentinel signs and symptoms are dark-coloured nasal septal (Fig. 6) or palatal ulcers or eschars (Figs. 7 and 8), fever, headache, nasal crusting, epistaxis, cough and mental changes [10]. There could also be skip lesions due to spread of the infection along the intima of blood vessels (Fig. 9 showing a tongue lesion in a patient of ALL with rhino-orbital mucormycosis).

Fig. 9 Skip mucor lesion on tongue (*arrow*) in patient with ALL and rhino-orbital mucormycosis

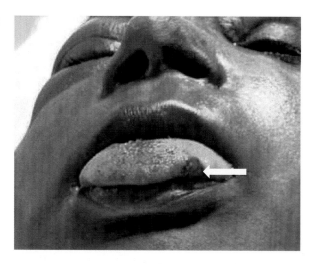

Tissue samples should ideally be taken from discoloured areas of the middle and inferior turbinate or septum under vision during a diagnostic nasal endoscopy.

Teaching point: *Samples taken from the nasal vestibule or swabs taken blindly do not help in the diagnosis and instead delay the diagnosis. The samples should be sent for both microbiological (KOH and fungal culture) and histopathological examination.*

- Decreased facial or nasal mucosal sensations may be present even in early stages of the disease before the development of other signs and symptoms.
- Gingival or palatal eschars or ulceration may be found (Figs. 7 and 8).

Ascioglu et al. [11] have suggested major and minor criteria for clinical diagnosis.

Minor criteria	Major criteria
Nasal discharge/stuffiness	Radiologic e/o sinus invasion, i.e. erosion of sinus walls, extension of infection to neighbouring structures, extensive skull base destruction
Nasal ulceration/eschar/epistaxis	
Periorbital swelling	
Maxillary tenderness	
Black necrotic lesions/perforation of palate	

Ophthalmic Examination

An ophthalmologist should assess the vision, field of vision and retinal pathology and look for ophthalmoplegia or chorioretinitis through the entire course of the patient's treatment.

Fig. 10 Oroantral fistula
(*black arrow*) in a diabetic
patient with chronic invasive
mucormycosis

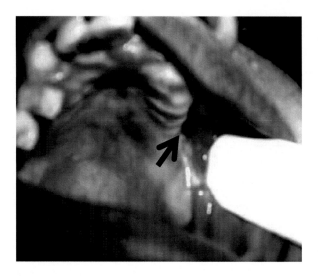

It has been recommended that nasal endoscopy and imaging studies are war-ranted if there is persistence of fever of unknown origin for more than 48 h despite appropriate antibiotic therapy and in the presence of localized sino-nasal symptoms in an immunocompromised patient [9, 12, 13].

Chronic Invasive Fungal Sinusitis

This usually develops in immunocompetent individuals but is also seen in diabetics and individuals with low level of immunocompromise [14]. There may be a history of chronic rhinosinusitis, and symptoms may consist of serosanguineous nasal dis-charge, epistaxis, nasal polyposis, fever or a persistent oroantral fistula (Fig. 10 and Fig. 8 in Chapter "Radiology in Invasive Fungal Sinusitis"). There could be devel-opment of sequestrum in the nose after several years (Figs. 11 and 12) or palatal ulcer (Fig. 13). The symptoms are persistent and recurrent and may take months and years to develop.

Chronic Invasive Granulomatous

This is usually seen in immunocompetent individuals and is usually caused by *Aspergillus flavus*. The presenting complaint is diplopia, and there may be proptosis in majority of the patients. There may be history of chronic rhinosinusitis.

Fig. 11 Nasal sequestrum (*arrow*) in a juvenile diabetic patient with chronic mucormycosis

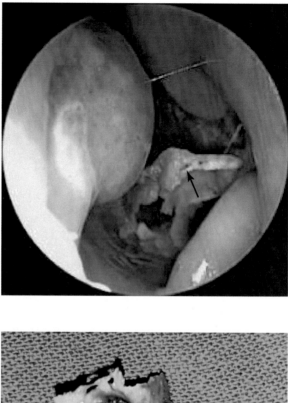

Fig. 12 Nasal sequestrum after removal from same patient as Fig. 11 in Chapter "Epidemiology, Pathogenesis, and Risk Factors"

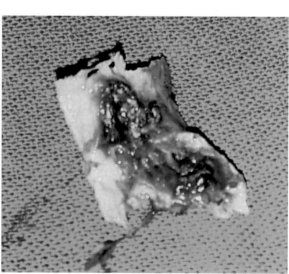

An algorithm for diagnosis of invasive fungal sinusitis and for diagnostic criteria is shown in Figs. 14 and Table 1, respectively.

Fig. 13 Palatal ulcer (*arrow*) in diabetic patient with chronic mucormycosis

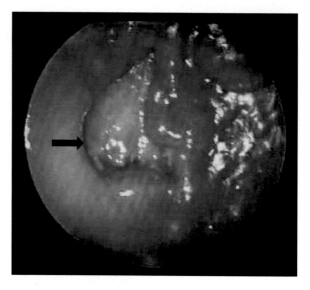

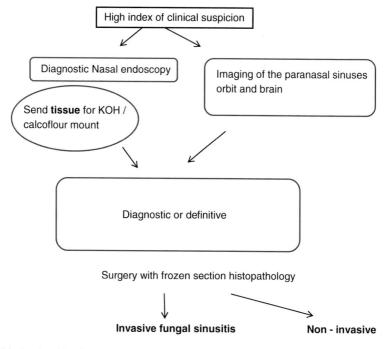

An Algorithm for diagnosis

High index of clinical suspicion

Diagnostic Nasal endoscopy

Send **tissue** for KOH / calcoflour mount

Imaging of the paranasal sinuses orbit and brain

Diagnostic or definitive

Surgery with frozen section histopathology

Invasive fungal sinusitis   **Non - invasive**

Fig. 14 An algorithm for diagnosis

Table 1 Diagnostic criteria for invasive fungal sinusitis [10]

1. Mucosal thickening or air fluid levels compatible with sinusitis on radiologic imaging
2. Histopathologic evidence of hyphal forms within sinus mucosa, submucosa, blood vessels or bone
3. Diagnosis of granulomatous invasive fungal sinusitis based on histopathologic evidence of hyphal forms within the sinus mucosa, submucosa, blood vessel or bone in association with granuloma containing giant cells. Concomitant stains for mycobacteria must be negative

References

1. Waitzman AA, Birt BD. Fungal sinusitis. J Otolaryngol. 1994;23(4):244–9.
2. Gillespie MB, O'Malley Jr BW, Francis HW. An approach to fulminant invasive fungal rhino-sinusitis in immunocompromised host. Arch Otolaryngol Head Neck Surg. 1998;124(5): 520–6.
3. Abramson E, Wilson D, Arky RA. Rhinocerebral phycomycosis in association with diabetic ketoacidosis. Ann Intern Med. 1967;66:735–42.
4. Epstein VA, Kern RC. Invasive fungal sinusitis and complications of rhinosinusitis. Otolaryngol Clin North Am. 2008;41:497–524.
5. Lehrer RI, Howard DH, Sypherd PS, et al. Mucormycosis. Ann Intern Med. 1980;93: 93–108.
6. Spellberg B, Edwards Jr J, Ibrahim A. Novel perspectives on mucormycosis: pathophysiology, presentation and management. Clin Microbiol Rev. 2005;18:556–69.
7. Talbot GH, Huang A, Provendar M. Invasive aspergillus rhinosinusitis in patients with acute leukemia. Rev Infect Dis. 1991;13:219–32.
8. Idris N, Lim LH. Nasal eschar: a warning sign of potentially fatal invasive fungal sinusitis in immunocompromised children. J Pediatr Hematol Oncol. 2012;34(4):e134–6.
9. Gillespie MB, O'Malley BW. An algorithmic approach to the diagnosis and management of invasive fungal rhinosinusitis in the immunocompromised patient. Otolaryngol Clin North Am. 2000;33(2):323–34.
10. DeShazo RD. Syndromes of invasive fungal sinusitis. Med Mycol. 2009;47(Suppl I):S 309–14.
11. Ascioglu S, Rex JH, de Pauw B, et al. Clinical infectious diseases. Clin Infect Dis. 2002;34(1):7–14. Epub 2001 Nov 26.
12. Ferguson BJ. Definitions of fungal rhinosinusitis. Otolaryngol Clin North Am. 2000;33(2): 227–35.
13. Park AH, Muntz HR, Smith ME, et al. Pediatric invasive fungal rhinosinusitis in immunocompromised children with cancer. Otolaryngol Head Neck Surg. 2005;133(3):411–6.
14. Aribandi M, McCoy VA, Bazan C. Imaging features of invasive and non-invasive fungal sinusitis: a review. Radiographics. 2007;27:1283–96.

Histopathology of Invasive Fungal Rhinosinusitis

R.B. Deshpande

Histopathological examination forms the basis of diagnosis, classification, and management of invasive fungal rhinosinusitis [1, 2]. In cases where fungal infection is suspected on clinical grounds, demonstration of fungal elements should be sufficient to start treatment, but histopathological examination is necessary to confirm the diagnosis of "invasive" fungal infection and to properly classify the fungal disease for further management.

Histopathological diagnosis of invasive fungal diseases has three components, namely, (a) demonstration of fungal elements (b) identifying tissue invasiveness, and (c) identifying type of inflammatory reaction – on the basis of which further classification is made.

In majority of the cases, fungal elements can be identified on hematoxylin and eosin (H&E)-stained sections. However, identification becomes easy with special staining techniques like periodic acid-Schiff (PAS) stain and Gomori's (Grocott–Gomori's) silver methenamine (GMS) preparation. Gomori methenamine has been described to be the most sensitive of the commonly used stains, and it has been recommended that a negative diagnosis should not be given unless a silver stain has been performed [3].

In both, PAS and GMS techniques, the principle is to demonstrate polysaccharide-rich fungal walls. In PAS staining, periodic acid oxidizes polysaccharides in to aldehydes which on reaction with Schiff's reagent produces purple or magenta color. Walls of fungal hyphae are stained magenta color highlighting the fungal structure.

In Grocott–Gomori's (or Gomori's) methenamine silver technique, the polysaccharides are oxidized in to pair of aldehydes. The aldehydes react with silver nitrate and reduce it in to metallic silver that deposits on the fungal wall making it stand out. In fact, GMS is not a stain in the strictest sense but causes silver deposition that makes the fungal elements more easily demonstrable.

R.B. Deshpande, MD
Department of Pathology, P.D. Hinduja Hospital,
Mahim, Mumbai, Maharashtra 400 016, India
e-mail: atharnas@yahoo.com

G. Mankekar (ed.), *Invasive Fungal Rhinosinusitis*,
DOI 10.1007/978-81-322-1530-1_5, © Springer India 2014

Both the PAS stain and GMS techniques are not specific for fungi. They only make the polysaccharide-rich fungal walls easily identifiable. There are many other structures in tissues – including collagen bands and vessel walls. To the uninitiated, these may look like fungal elements. Fungi are identified by their structural characteristics and not on positive or negative staining.

Invasiveness of the disease is determined by the presence of the fungal elements in the submucosa, invasion into the vessel walls and the lumen with consequent vascular thrombosis, and infarction of the tissue. While in the chronic disease, there is predominantly chronic inflammatory cell component or there is granulomatous reaction.

Based on the type of inflammatory reaction and temporal profile of the pathologic process, invasive fungal rhinosinusitis is divided in to three groups:

(a) Acute fulminant invasive rhinosinusitis
(b) Chronic invasive fungal rhinosinusitis
(c) Chronic granulomatous rhinosinusitis

Acute Fulminant Invasive Fungal Rhinosinusitis

This occurs mainly in patients with immunosuppression, or ketoacidosis of diabetes mellitus, or uremia of chronic renal disease but is also being reported in immunocompetent patients. The fungi most often involved are *Mucor* species or *Aspergillus*. There is usually little or no appreciable inflammatory cell reaction. Fungal hyphae invade the tissue especially the vessel walls, resulting in thrombosis of the vessels and consequent infarction of the tissue. Both invasive mucormycosis and aspergillosis have an affinity for invading blood vessels [4–7] (Fig. 1). In particular, invasive Mucor has a strong affinity for arteries. Histopathological features include growth along the internal elastic lamina that results in dissection away from the media, as well as growth into the blood vessel lumen, producing endothelial damage and initiating thrombosis [8] (Fig. 2).

These fungi, having once invaded the vessels, disseminate rapidly in fulminant fashion, extending to intracranial spaces, carotid artery, etc. and prove fatal in a very short time. Rapid diagnosis and prompt treatment may save at least some of these patients.

Histopathologists involved in diagnosis of such cases should be alerted to the possibility of acute invasive fungal infection. Intraoperative frozen section examination may save considerable time in diagnosis. If intraoperative frozen section examination facility is not available and if the primary physician/surgeon communicates to the pathologist of the clinical suspicion of invasive fungal sinusitis, then routine processing may be done in rapid fashion and the result promptly communicated to the treating physician without delay.

Once the possibility of fungal infection is considered, frozen section diagnosis should not be difficult. Vascular invasion, infarction of the tissue, and presence of fungi are not difficult to identify. Fungi can be identified even on Toluidine blue stain or H&E staining. Mucor species which is most often involved in acute

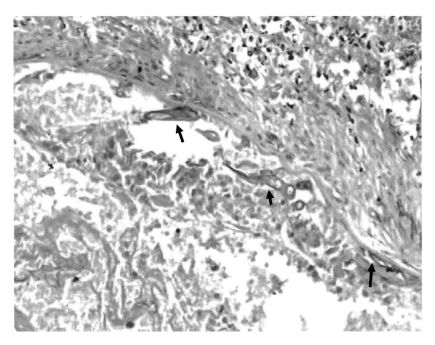

Fig. 1 PAS-stained sections showing broad aseptate fungal hyphae (*arrows*) infiltrating the vessel wall causing a thrombus

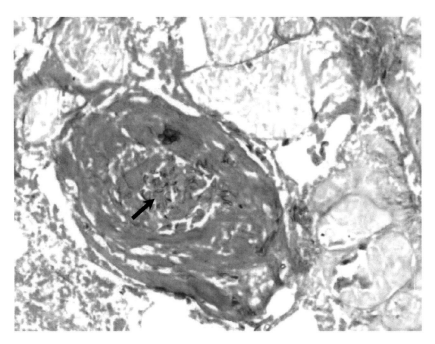

Fig. 2 PAS-stained section showing infarcted adipose tissue with broad aseptate fungal hyphae (*arrow*) infiltrating into the lumen on the vessel causing thrombus

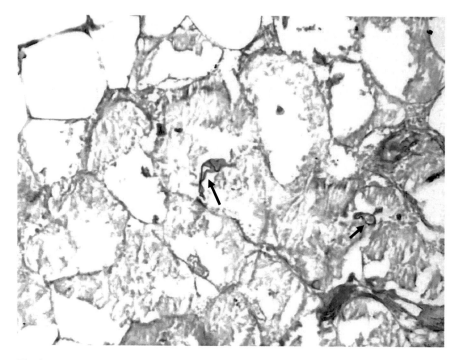

Fig. 3 H&E stain, original magnification 400× showing infarcted fat tissue with broad aseptate fungal hyphae (*arrows*) folding on themselves with characteristic features of mucormycosis

fulminant processes can be identified by broad (10–15 μm wide) ribbon-like aseptate fungal hyphae which fold on themselves and branch at right angles (Figs. 3, 4, and 5), while Aspergillus species which also may cause acute invasive fulminant process (Figs. 8 and 9) appears as narrow (2–5 μm wide) septate acutely branching fungal hyphae (Figs. 7 and 8).

Chronic Invasive Fungal Rhinosinusitis (Fig. 6)

In these cases, there is usually destruction of the tissue with chronic abscess-like inflammatory reaction with presence of fungal elements within the exudate. There is usually nothing – either clinically or histologically to alert the pathologist about the possibility of fungal etiology and hence the diagnosis may be missed. Constant alertness and a high level of suspicion of fungal etiology in all such cases irrespective of the underlying disorders helps in identifying such cases. Unlike the neutrophil-rich, highly necrotic, and angiotrophic process seen in acute invasive fungal sinusitis, there is a low-grade mixed cellular infiltrate in affected tissues [9]. Usually this occurs in diabetics, is slowly progressive, and elicits limited inflammation.

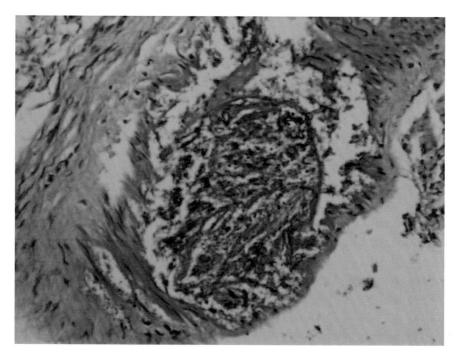

Fig. 4 H&E stain (original magnification 400×) fungal hyphae of Mucor in thrombosed blood vessel

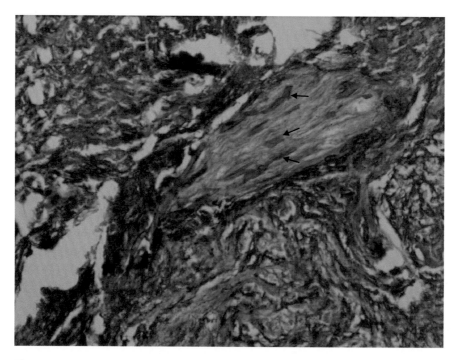

Fig. 5 H&E stain (original magnification 400×) showing fungal hyphae of Mucor (*arrows*) in vascular lumen

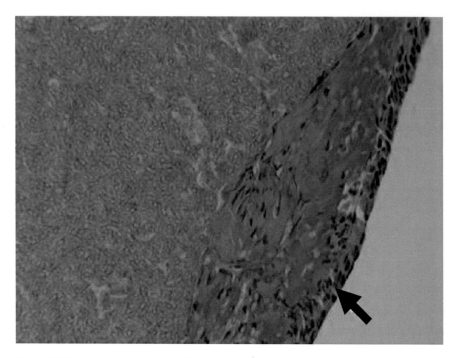

Fig. 6 H&E stain showing chronic inflammatory exudate with fungi (*arrow*) within the exudate

Chronic Granulomatous Fungal Rhinosinusitis

Other terms for this condition include "indolent fungal sinusitis" and primary paranasal granuloma. Published cases include those from Sudan (due to *Aspergillus flavus*) and St Louis, MO [10, 11]. Patients invariably have no predisposing factors, and the lesion usually presents as a destructive process raising the suspicion of malignancy. There is often destructive growth eroding in to the orbit. Histologically this presents as chronic granulomatous process with non-necrotizing granuloma composed of clusters or sheets of foreign-body-type multinucleated giant cells with fair number of eosinophils in the background. The combination of sheets/ clusters of foreign-body-type multinucleated giant cells with eosinophils in the background should be enough to alert the pathologist about possibility of fungal (mainly *Aspergillus flavus*) disease. Close look at the giant cells even in frozen sections or paraffin sections stained with hematoxylin and eosin stain should reveal short well-stained or shadow-like unstained fungal hyphae in the cytoplasm of the giant cells (Fig. 7). GMS stain (Fig. 8) and PAS stain (Fig. 9) also reveal the characteristic features of the fungus within the giant cells. Tuberculosis does not commonly involve the paranasal sinuses. Also concomitant stains for mycobacteria are negative. Hence, any granulomatous disease causing destruction of bone that initially clinically presents as a malignancy in young immunocompetent patients should alert the pathologist to the possibility of chronic invasive granulomatous sinusitis.

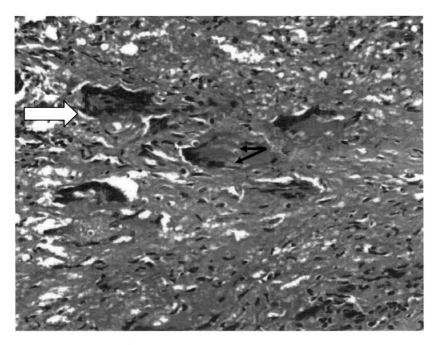

Fig. 7 H&E stain (original magnification 400×) showing clusters of multinucleate foreign-body-type giant cells (*broad white arrow*) with negatively stained fungal hyphae (*thin black arrows*)

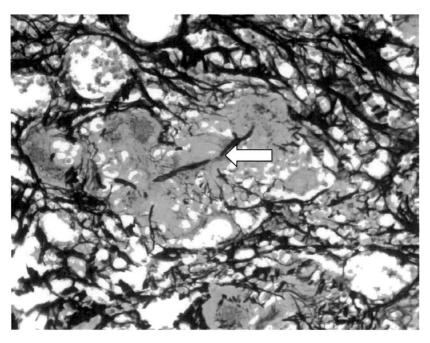

Fig. 8 Gomori's methenamine silver impregnated for fungus showing septate branching fungal hyphae in the giant cells. Note that the collagen surrounding the giant cells are also stained black. Fungi are identified by their septate and branching features (*white arrow*)

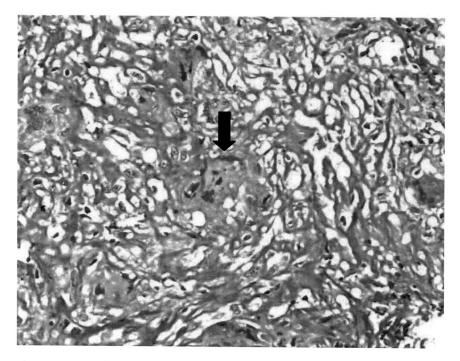

Fig. 9 PAS-stained sections showing septate branching fungal hyphae (*black arrow*) in the giant cell. Surrounding collagen is also stained pink

In all these cases, fungal etiology is missed by the inexperienced pathologist not because of the difficulty in identifying the fungi histologically but because of the lack of awareness of this possibility. Clinicians who suspect fungal etiology should make it a point to discuss the case with the concerned pathologist personally. Acute invasive fungal rhinosinusitis is one of the most critical emergency situations for the pathologists. Diagnosis in such cases should be rapid with prompt communication to the treating physician of the diagnosis.

The pathologist should also be able to identify noninvasive fungal sinusitis and differentiate it from the invasive variety. Noninvasive fungal rhinosinusitis includes "fungal ball" and allergic fungal sinusitis (AFS). These have characteristic histopathological appearance with absence of fungal invasion of the tissues.

Fungal Ball

In these cases, histopathology shows multitude of pale fungal hyphae compressed in the center, with appearance of morphology at the periphery

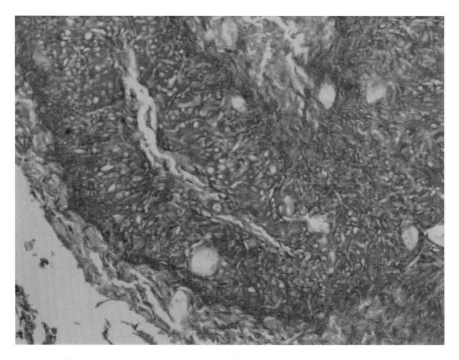

Fig. 10 H&E stain (original magnification 400×) showing compactly packed septate branching fungal hyphae morphologically resembling *Aspergillus* spp. indicative of fungal ball

(Fig. 10). The surrounding mucosa usually shows dense mixed inflammatory infiltrate.

Allergic Fungal Sinusitis (Fig. 11a, b)

The diagnosis of AFS is primarily histopathological although there are clinical and radiological features to distinguish it from invasive fungal sinusitis. Characteristic allergic mucin is seen on H&E stains as strongly staining laminated concretions of pyknotic and degranulated eosinophils surrounded by areas of lightly staining mucin sprinkled with Charcot–Leyden crystals [12–14]. Staining of allergic mucin with fungal stains like Gomori's (GMS) may show scattered fungal hyphae within the allergic mucin [12–16]. There is no evidence of mucosal fungal invasion, including features of tissue invasion like mucosal necrosis, granuloma formation, or giant cells. An important fact to remember is that allergic mucin without fungal involvement can be seen in patients with the non-AFS "eosinophilic mucin rhinosinusitis" [17, 18].

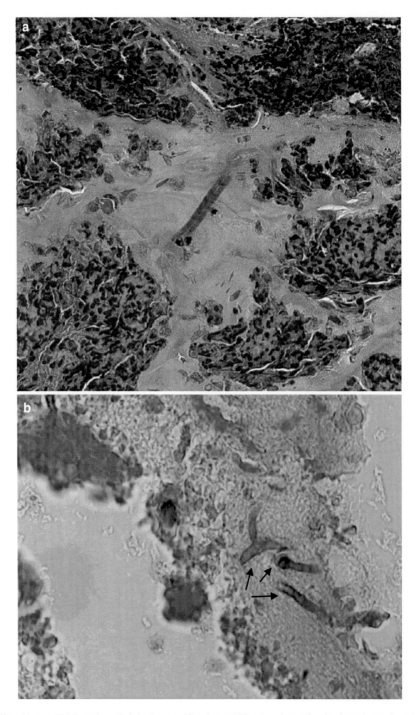

Fig. 11 (**a**) H&E stain. (Original magnification ×400) showing allergic fungal mucin with Charcot–Leyden crystals. (**b**) PAS stain (original magnification ×400) showing allergic mucin with septate fungal hyphae (*arrows*)

References

1. deShazo RD, O'Brien M, Chapin K, et al. A new classification and diagnostic criteria for invasive fungal sinusitis. Arch Otolaryngol Head Neck Surg. 1997;123:1181–8.
2. Das A, Bal A, Chakarabarti A, Panda N, Joshi K. Spectrum of fungal rhinosinusitis; a histopathologist's perspective. Histopathology. 2009;54:854–9.
3. Schell WA. Histopathology of fungal rhinosinusitis. Otolaryngol Clin North Am. 2000;33:251–76.
4. Barnes L, Peel RL. Head and neck pathology: a text/atlas of differential diagnosis. New York: Igahu-Shoin; 1990. p. 170.
5. Michaels L. Ear, nose and throat histopathology. New York: Springer; 1987. p. 146–8.
6. Johnson JT. Infections. In: Cummings CW, Krause CJ, editors. Otolaryngology head neck surgery, vol. 2. 2nd ed. St. Louis: Mosby Year Book; 1993. p. 931–3.
7. Myerowitz RL, Guggenheimer J, Barnes L. Infectious diseases of the head and neck. New York: Marcel Dekker; 1985. p. 1784–6.
8. Straatsma BR, Zimmerman LE, Gass JDM. Phycomycosis: a clinicopathologic study of fifty one cases. Lab Invest. 1962;11:963–85.
9. Milro CM, Blanshard JD, Lucas S, Michaels L. Aspergillosis of the nose and paranasal sinuses. J Clin Pathol. 1989;42:123–7.
10. Veress B, Malik OA, el-Tayeb AA, et al. Further observations on the primary paranasal *Aspergillosis* granuloma in the Sudan: a morphological study of 46 cases. Am J Trop Med Hyg. 1973;22:765–72.
11. Currens J, Hutcheson PS, Slavin RG, Citardi MJ. Primary paranasal *Aspergillus* granuloma: a case report and review of literature. Am J Rhinol. 2002;16:165–8.
12. Schubert MS, Goetz DW. Evaluation and treatment of allergic fungal sinusitis. I. Demographics and diagnosis. J Allergy Clin Immunol. 1998;102:387–94.
13. Katzenstein AA, Sale SR, Greenburger PA. Allergic *Aspergillus* sinusitis: a newly recognized form of sinusitis. J Allergy Clin Immunol. 1983;72:89–93.
14. Gourley DS, Whisman BA, Jorgensen NL, et al. Allergic *Bipolaris* sinusitis. Clinical and histopathological characteristics. J Allergy Clin Immunol. 1990;85:583–91.
15. Bent III JP, Kuhn FA. Diagnosis of allergic fungal sinusitis. Otolaryngol Head Neck Surg. 1994;111:580–8.
16. de Shazo RD, Swain RE. Diagnostic criteria for allergic fungal sinusitis. J Allergy Clin Immunol. 1995;95:24–35.
17. Ferguson BJ. Eosinophilic mucin rhinosinusitis: a distinct clinicopathological entity. Laryngoscope. 2000;110:799–813.
18. Ramadan HH, Quraishi HA. Allergic mucin sinusitis without fungus. Am J Rhinol. 1997;11: 145–7.

Microbiology in Invasive Fungal Sinusitis

Anjali Shetty and Camilla Rodrigues

Introduction

In the past few decades, the incidence of invasive fungal rhinosinusitis cases in tertiary care centers has been steadily increasing with the gradual increase in the number of immunocompromised patients. India contributes to about 40 % of the global burden of zygomycosis [1]. Fungal spores are ubiquitous and are continuously being inhaled, leading to colonization of the sinuses. This colonization may lead to chronic sinusitis and occasionally invasive fungal infection especially in an immunocompromised host.

Fungi are eukaryotes (possess nuclear membrane), depend on an external source for nutrition, and may consist of hyphal segments or unicellular organisms. Fungal infections were a rarity in the past with the predominant problem being allergy, mycotoxicoses from ingested toxins, and mushroom poisoning.

There are four main groups (phyla) of true fungi—*Ascomycota, Basidiomycota, Zygomycota*, and Deuteromycota (Fungi imperfecti). Ascomycota include dermatophytes, *Aspergillus* spp., *Histoplasma capsulatum, and Blastomyces dermatitidis*. The most common fungal infections are caused by dermatophytes, fungi that colonize dead keratinized tissue including skin, finger, and toenails. Dermatophytes cause superficial infections such as "ringworm" that are unsightly and difficult to treat, but rarely serious. *Aspergillus fumigatus*, one of the most important of these opportunists, produces small, airborne spores that are frequently inhaled; in some individuals, the fungus starts growing invasively, causing a disease known as aspergillosis, especially in immunocompromised individuals.

A. Shetty, MRCP, FRCPath (✉) • C. Rodrigues, MD
Department of Microbiology, P.D. Hinduja Hospital,
Mahim, Mumbai, Maharashtra 400 016, India
e-mail: anjalishettyuk@yahoo.co.uk;
dr_crodrigues@hindujahospital.com

G. Mankekar (ed.), *Invasive Fungal Rhinosinusitis*,
DOI 10.1007/978-81-322-1530-1_6, © Springer India 2014

Mucormycosis is the common term used to describe infections caused by fungi belonging to the order Mucorales. Zygomycosis, a term which was used earlier to describe these life-threatening infections, has become less accurate based on a recent taxonomic reclassification (based on molecular identification) that abolished Zygomycetes as a class [2, 3].

Mucormycosis and entomophthoramycosis were earlier encompassed by the term zygomycosis. Changes in taxonomy due to molecular phylogenetic analyses have, however, led to the class name Zygomycota being replaced by Glomeromycota. In the current classification, the agents of mucormycosis have been placed under the subphylum Mucormycotina, and the agents of Entomophthoramycosis are now in the subphylum Entomophthoramycotina. Since the phylum Zygomycota does not exist any longer, the disease name zygomycosis has become obsolete.

Mucorales includes *Rhizopus* spp., *Absidia* spp., *Rhizomucor* spp., *and Mucor* spp. These organisms can cause rhinocerebral, pulmonary, gastrointestinal, cutaneous, or disseminated infection in the immunosuppressed host and account for up to 75 % of mucormycosis cases encountered in hematologic malignancy patients [4]. Entomophthoramycosis includes infections due to *Conidiobolus* spp. *and Basidiobolus* spp. They are often seen in tropical environment causing infections of the paranasal sinuses and subcutaneous tissues. These infections are seen in immunocompetent individuals and have a chronic course. *Conidiobolus* spp. affects the head and face. Subcutaneous rhinofacial infection is the most common presentation. Symptoms include nasal discharge, unilateral nasal obstruction, sinus tenderness, and facial swelling (Fig. 1). Basidiobolus spp. involves the subcutaneous tissues of the trunk and arms.

Basidiomycota includes *Cryptococcus neoformans*. This organism is an encapsulated yeast which can cause disease in immunocompetent individuals as well as immunosuppressed patients. Infection occurs following inhalation and meningitis is the most common presentation.

Deuteromycota (Fungi imperfecti) includes *Candida* spp., *Coccidioides immitis, and Sporothrix schenckii. Candida* species can cause both superficial and invasive infections. It is also part of the normal flora of the gastrointestinal tract.

Fungi isolated in invasive fungal rhinosinusitis while showing geographic variation are often similar in particular forms of fungal disease [5]. For example, *A. fumigatus, A. flavus, and Rhizopus* sp. are uniformly seen in patients with acute invasive disease worldwide [6–8].

Acute Invasive Fungal Rhinosinusitis

Two distinct patient populations are seen [9]: one group of patients is patients with diabetes, especially with diabetic ketoacidosis and second group with neutropenia. Up to 80 % of invasive fungal infections in the first group are caused by fungi belonging to the order Zygomycetes such *as Rhizopus* sp., *Rhizomucor* sp., *Absidia* sp., *and Mucor* sp. [10]. This disease is more rapidly progressive with high

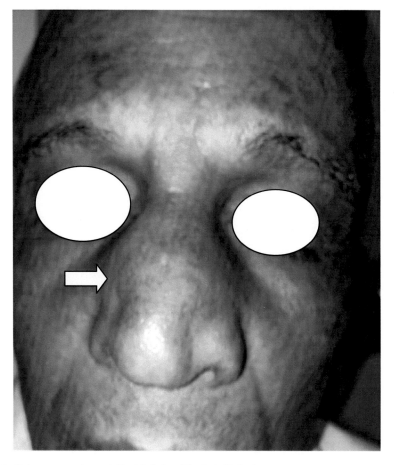

Fig. 1 Subcutaneous (*arrow*) Conidiobolus rhinofacial infection

mortality and morbidity probably due to the high virulence of these fungi as well as due to diagnosis of the disease at a late stage [9].

The other group is immunocompromised patients with severe neutropenia, e.g., patients with hematologic malignancies; patients undergoing chemotherapy or systemic steroid therapy or bone, organ, or stem cell transplantation; or patients with AIDS. Aspergillus species is responsible for up to 80 % of infections in this group [10]. In India, *A. flavus* [11] is the most common (80 %) while in the Middle East, *A. fumigatus* [12] is the most common (50 %) causative agent. Nasal septal ulceration has also been described with Fusarium species and *Pseudallescheria boydii*.

Among the zygomycotic species causing IFS, *Rhizopus arrhizus* is the most frequent agent followed by *Rhizopus microsporus*, *Absidia corymbifera*, *Rhizomucor pusillus*, and *Mucor circinelloides* [13, 14]. Another agent, *Apophysomyces elegans*, is also responsible for zygomycosis in India [1]. Sridhara et al. [15] have reported an increasing trend of mucormycosis in immunocompetent individuals. Three out of eight immunocompetent cases reported by them were infected by *Apophysomyces elegans* [15].

Wueppenhorst et al. [16] have reported a case of fulminant invasive fungal sinusitis caused by *Conidiobolus incongruus* in Germany. They concluded that diagnostics relying exclusively on histopathological findings could misdiagnose entomophthoramycosis as mucormycosis, and therefore, species identification is indispensable for collection of data for the adequate treatment of the condition.

Chronic Invasive Fungal Rhinosinusitis

Aspergillus species, dematiaceous molds such as *Bipolaris*, *Curvularia*, and *Pseudallescheria boydii* are the fungi implicated in this disease. *Aspergillus fumigatus* is the most commonly isolated fungus [17] although *Mucor* sp. is also known to be a causative agent especially in diabetics.

Chronic Granulomatous Rhinosinusitis

Aspergillus flavus is the fungus most often implicated in this disease. Paranasal granuloma is a peculiar syndrome associated with proptosis that has also been called indolent fungal sinusitis in immune competent persons. The fungus *A. flavus* shows exuberant growth with regional tissue invasion, non-caseating granulomas, giant cells, and plasma cells. This condition is known to occur in Saudi Arabia, Sudan, India, and Pakistan [11, 18]. This is rarely seen in the USA [19].

Diagnosis

Specimen – Tissue samples or aspirates are recommended as opposed to swabs as the material obtained in tissue and aspirate is much more than in swabs, thus increasing the yield.

Microscopy

KOH Wet Mount

Potassium hydroxide digests proteinaceous material and debris and allows visualization of the fungal hyphae under a light microscope (Fig. 2).

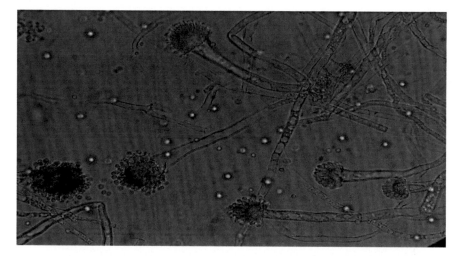

Fig. 2 KOH mount of *Aspergillus*

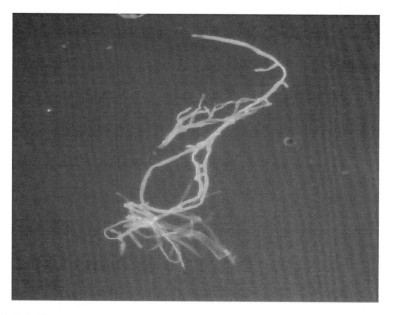

Fig. 3 Calcofluor preparation of aseptate fungal filaments

Calcofluor Staining

It is difficult to stain fungi with routine stains, but this stain binds to the chitin and cellulose in the fungal cell wall and demonstrates bright green to blue fluorescence under a fluorescent microscope making it easier to demonstrate the fungi (Figs. 3 and 4). Sensitivity increased by 15 % in demonstrating fungal hyphae when

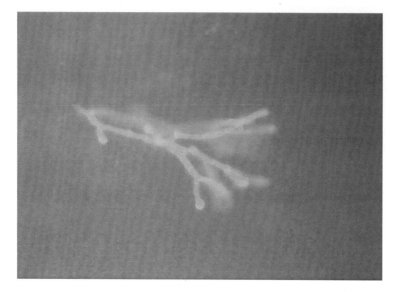

Fig. 4 Calcofluor preparation of septate fungi

calcofluor white was added to KOH wet mounts in a Chinese study on fungal keratitis [22]. For rapid diagnosis, clinicians should request for calcofluor/KOH mount.

Lactophenol cotton blue is a widely used method of staining and observing fungi (Figs. 5a, b and 6). On microscopy one can comment on the presence or absence of septae. Aseptate fungi are Mucorales (Fig. 3). Septate fungi are *Aspergillus* sp., *Fusarium* spp., *Scedosporium* spp., etc. (Fig. 4). *Aspergillus* spp. demonstrates acute angle branching and Mucorales demonstrates right angle branching. Practically, it may be difficult to comment on the branching pattern.

Culture

Fungal culture is difficult and often no growth is achieved. Fungal culture specimens should be obtained preferably before starting antifungal therapy. Initiation of antifungals prior to culture reduces the chances of growing fungus on culture. While processing the sample for culture, it is important to remember that grinding and freeze-thawing of the specimen will lead to a decreased yield of Mucorales.

The samples are cultured on agar such as Sabouraud dextrose agar (Figs. 7, 8, 9, 10 and 11), brain-heart infusion agar, etc. with antibiotics. The agar is incubated at both room temperature and 37 °C. Macroscopic and microscopic examination of cultures aids in the diagnosis of fungus. Fungal cultures should be examined biweekly for a period of 4 weeks before they are declared as negative.

Fig. 5 (**a**) Lactophenol cotton *blue* preparation of *Aspergillus fumigatus*. (**b**) LCB preparation of *Aspergillus fumigatus* head

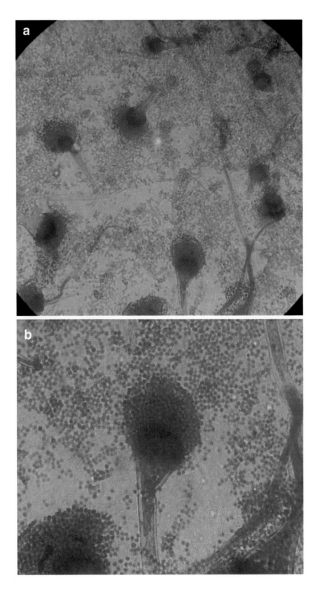

Fig. 6 Lactophenol cotton *blue* preparation of *Rhizopus* spp

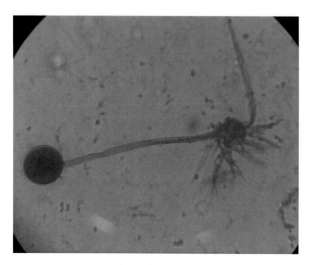

Fig. 7 *Aspergillus fumigatus* on Sabouraud dextrose agar (SDA)

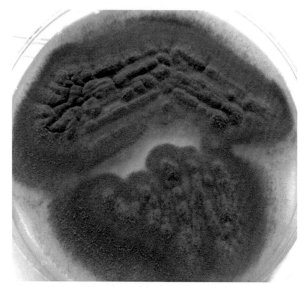

Aspergillus Galactomannan

This is a noninvasive test to diagnose invasive aspergillosis. It detects galactomannan, which is a polysaccharide cell wall component that is released by *Aspergillus* spp. during hyphal growth. The latex test had poor sensitivity and has been largely replaced by a double sandwich ELISA. FDA cutoff for this test is 0.5 ng/ml, though

Fig. 8 Mucor on Sabouraud dextrose agar

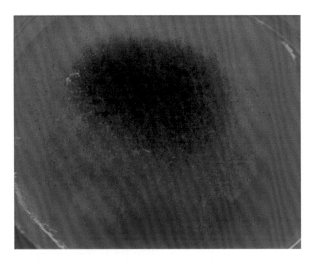

Fig. 9 *Aspergillus flavus* on Sabourad dextrose agar

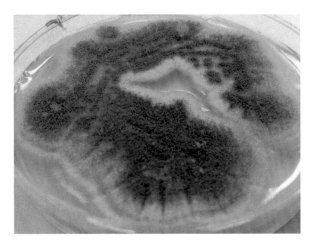

studies use different cutoffs of positivity. Together with host factors and clinical criteria, a positive serum galactomannan test would suggest probable invasive aspergillosis [1]. This test has shown variable sensitivity and specificity and is impacted by prior antifungal therapy. False positivity is known to occur due to the use of piperacillin-tazobactam and also in children. Cross reaction occurs with other fungi such as *Paecilomyces* spp., *Alternaria* spp., *Penicillium* spp., etc. A study in patients with hematological malignancy in Taiwan [21] had 16 patients with invasive fungal sinusitis who had serial follow-up of Aspergillus galactomannan. Sensitivity was 64 % and specificity was 60 % for the diagnosis of invasive aspergillus sinusitis when compared to the EORTC criteria [22].

Fig. 10 *Scedosporium* on
SDA

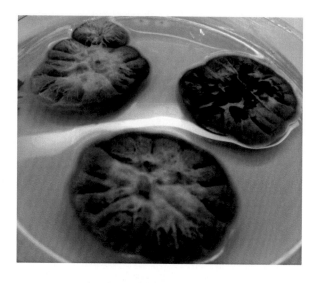

Fig. 11 *A. fumigatus* on
CZA (Czapek's agar)

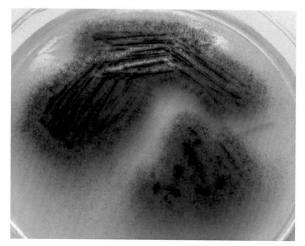

References

1. Chakrabarti A, Chatterjee SS, Shivaprakash MR. Overview of opportunistic fungal infections in India. J Med Mycol. 2008;49:165–72.
2. Spellberg B, Edwards Jr J, Ibrahim A. Novel perspectives on mucormycosis: pathophysiology, presentation and management. Clin Microbiol Rev. 2005;18(3):556–69.
3. Kontoyiannis DP, Lewis RE. Agents of mucormycosis and related species. In: Mandell GL, Bennett JE, Dolin R, editors. Principles and practice of infectious diseases, vol. 2. 6th ed. Philadelphia: Elsevier Churchill Livingstone; 2005. p. 2973.
4. Kontoyiannis DP, Lionakis MS, Lewis RE, et al. Zygomycosis in a tertiary care center in the era of Aspergillus active antifungal therapy: a case control observational study of 27 recent cases. J Infect Dis. 2005;191(8):1350–60.

5. Montone KT, Livolski VA, Feldman MD, et al. Fungal rhinosinusitis: a retrospective microbiologic and pathologic review of 400 patients at a single university medical center. Indian J Otolaryngol. 2012. doi:10.1155/2012/684835.
6. Das A, Bal A, Chakrabarti A, et al. Spectrum of fungal rhinosinusitis: histopathologist's perspective. Histopathology. 2009;54(7):854–9.
7. Panda NK, Sharma SC, Chakrabarti A, et al. Paranasal sinus mycosis in north India. Mycoses. 1998;41(7–8):281–6.
8. Challa S, Uppin SG, Hanumanthu A, et al. Fungal rhinosinusitis: a clinicopathological study from South India. Eur Arch Otorhinolaryngol. 2010;267(8):1239–45.
9. Aribandi M, McCoy VA, Bazan C. Imaging features of invasive and non-invasive fungal sinusitis. A review. Radiographics. 2007;27:1283–96.
10. Gillespie MB, O'Malley Jr BW, Francis HW. An approach to fulminant invasive fungal rhinosinusitis in the immunocompromised host. Arch Otolaryngol Head Neck Surg. 1998;124(5):520–6.
11. Chakrabarti A, Sharma SC, Chander J. Epidemiology and pathogenesis of paranasal sinus mycoses. Otolaryngol Head Neck Surg. 1992;107:745–50.
12. Taj-Aldeen SJ, Hilal AA, Schell WA. Allergic fungal rhinosinusitis: a report of 8 cases. Am J Otolaryngol. 2004;25:213–8.
13. Diwakar A, Dewan RK, Chowdhury A, et al. Zygomycosis – a case report and overview of the disease in India. Mycoses. 2007;50:247–54.
14. Chakrabarti A, Das A, Mandal J, et al. The rising trend of invasive zygomycosis in patients with uncontrolled diabetes mellitus. Med Mycol. 2006;44:335–42.
15. Sridhara SR, Paragache G, Panda NK, Chakrabarti A. Mucormycosis in immunocompetent individuals: an increasing trend. J Otolaryngol. 2005;34(6):402–6.
16. Wueppenhorst N, Lee M-K, Rapplod E, Kayser G, Beckervordersandforth J, de With K, Serr A. Rhino-orbito-cerebral zygomycosis caused by Conidiobolus incongruous in an immunocompromised patient in Germany. J Clin Microbiol. 2010;48(11):4322–5. doi: 10.1128/ JCM.01188-10. Epub 2010 Sep 22.
17. deShazo RD,Chapin K, Swain R. Fungal sinusitis. N Eng J Med. 1997; 337:254–59.
18. Hussain S, Salahuddin N, Ahmad I, et al. Rhinocerebral invasive mycosis: occurrence in immunocompetent individuals. Eur J Radiol. 1995;20:151–5.
19. Washburn RG, Kennedy DW, Begley MG, et al. Chronic fungal sinusitis in apparently normal hosts. Medicine. 1988;67:231–47.
20. Weihong Z, Huashan Y, Lili J, Lei H, Liya W. The journal of international medical research. 2010 38:1961–7
21. Chien-Yuan C, Wang-Huei S, Aristine C, Yee-chun C, Woie T, Jih-Luh T, et al. Invasive fungal sinusitis in patients with hematological malignancy: 15 years experience in a single university hospital in Taiwan. BMC Infect Dis. 2011;11:250. 1–9.
22. De Pauw B, Walsh TJ, Donnelly JP, Stevens DA, Edwards JE, Calandra Y, European Organization of Research and Treatment of Cancer/Invasive Fungal Infections Cooperative Group; National Institute of Allergy and Infectious Diseases Mycoses Study Group (EORTC/ MSG) Consensus Group, et al. Revised definitions of invasive fungal disease. Clin Infect Dis. 2008;46:1813–21.

Radiology in Invasive Fungal Sinusitis

Santosh Gupta and Shailendra Maheshwari

Although the diagnosis of invasive fungal sinusitis is based on histopathological evidence, imaging is important in patients in whom complicated sinusitis is suspected, especially in the absence of the specific clinical signs and symptoms suggestive of invasive fungal sinusitis. In such difficult to manage situations, imaging with its ability to detect subtle evidence of invasive disease has a crucial role in management [1] and helps in early diagnosis. The radiologist can alert the clinician by identifying the different types of fungal sinusitis from their distinct radiologic features, which would enable the physician to decide appropriate management techniques. This chapter discusses the radiological characteristics of both invasive and noninvasive sinusitis to enable the clinician to differentiate between the types.

Plain radiographs and tomograms of paranasal sinuses focused primarily on multifocal bone destruction as an aid to the diagnosis of invasive fungal sinusitis and in the evaluation of advanced disease [1, 2]. These conventional radiological techniques are now obsolete especially with the advent of cross-sectional imaging. Usually CT scan is the primary imaging modality used to evaluate paranasal sinuses in general, and so also it tends to be the first imaging modality requested for by the clinicians, in patients suspected to have invasive fungal sinusitis. The scan can serve as a baseline examination to determine a potential source for the fever experienced by severely neutropenic or immunocompromised patients with sinusitis. Some institutions and clinicians may prefer MR imaging for the initial evaluation of patients with complicated sinusitis. MR imaging is better able to depict advanced disease involving the orbit or brain, extra axial space and meninges, and the cavernous sinuses [3]. Advantages of CT are quick examination, therefore better patient compliance, better depiction of bony erosions/destruction, and ease of availability. Disadvantages of CT are lack of soft tissue resolution, difficulty in seeing extent especially intracranial and soft tissue planes, and problems of radiation.

S. Gupta, MD (✉) • S. Maheshwari, DNB, DMRD
Department of Radiology, PD Hinduja Hospital and MRC,
Mahim, Mumbai, Maharashtra, India
e-mail: drsantoshgupta@gmail.com

G. Mankekar (ed.), *Invasive Fungal Rhinosinusitis*,
DOI 10.1007/978-81-322-1530-1_7, © Springer India 2014

51

Advantage of MRI is very good soft tissue resolution, therefore shows extent including complications such as intracranial extension, vascular and soft tissue involvement far better, and lack of any radiation. Also advanced imaging such as perfusion/diffusion can be used with MRI, although these are still in research.

Disadvantages of MRI are long duration of procedure (which can be a problem in uncooperative patients, and they may require sedation), cost of MRI test (which is still an issue for many patients in countries like India), and lack of easy availability or accessibility.

CT Technique: Usually a limited CT of paranasal sinuses is a direct coronal CT, obtained with patient in prone position, which is reviewed in both soft tissue and bone window setting algorithm. In case of clinical suspicion of invasive fungal sinusitis, one may perform a dedicated, plain as well as post-contrast helical CT in supine position, followed by coronal reformation. Contrast study may be performed especially if there are no MRI facilities available. Ideal situation would be to do a simple limited plain coronal CT, followed by MRI.

MRI technique:

Dedicated MRI of paranasal sinuses includes coronal and axial T1 and coronal and axial STIR/T2 fat sat, followed by post-gadolinium-enhanced coronal and axial T1 fat-sat sequences. Pre- and post-contrast brain screening sequences must be a part of the protocol. Additional sequences such as perfusion, diffusion, and MR spectroscopy may be performed as and when needed.

According to de Shazo et al. [4], there are three distinct entities of invasive fungal sinusitis with their specific clinical and radiologic features: acute invasive, chronic invasive, and chronic granulomatous. In addition, the noninvasive types include allergic fungal rhinosinusitis and fungal ball.

Acute Invasive Fungal Sinusitis

This is usually caused by fungi belonging to the order Zygomycetes such *as Rhizopus* sp., *Rhizomucor* sp., *Absidia* sp., *and Mucor* sp. or Aspergillus species. On CT imaging, acute invasive fungal sinusitis in the initial stage may show minimal mucosal thickening or relatively small soft tissue in the nasal cavity and ethmoid or sphenoid sinus (Fig. 1). Obliteration and stranding in the peri-antral fat is a subtle sign of such extension and must be looked for in all patients at risk for acute invasive fungal sinusitis [3] (Figs. 2 and 3). Possible theories have been propounded to explain early peri-antral soft tissue infiltration prior to bone changes in invasive fungal sinusitis [3] – propensity of these fungi to initiate thrombosis could result in vascular congestion, in which case, the peri-antral soft tissue infiltration may be that of peri-antral "edema"; alternatively, the peri-antral soft tissue infiltration could represent the presence of fungal elements outside the maxillary sinus, which may be explained by the tendency these fungi have to spread along blood vessels. Direct spread through the perivascular spaces into the peri-antral fat could account for the peri-antral soft tissue infiltration beyond the confines of the bony maxilla. Acute

Fig. 1 Coronal CT shows soft tissue opacification of the left ethmoid and maxillary sinuses. Note subtle irregularity of adjacent left lamina papyracea with minimal intraorbital fat stranding, suggesting acute invasive fungal sinusitis

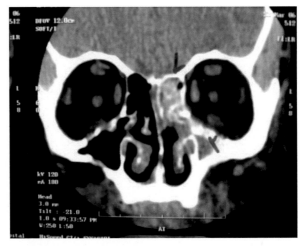

Fig. 2 MRI axial T1 image shows left peri-antral fat stranding (*arrow*), which may be an early sign of invasive fungal sinusitis

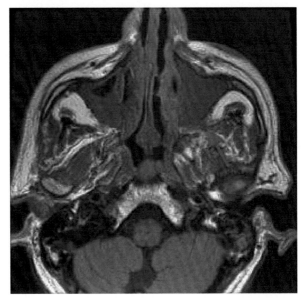

invasive has a predilection for unilateral involvement of the ethmoid and sphenoid sinuses [5, 6]. Radiological diagnosis can be difficult at this stage as the intra-sinus soft tissue or mucosal thickening may be minimal and not very obvious, and in addition the bone erosion may be very subtle. As the invasive fungi tend to spread along the blood vessels, the bony walls of the sinuses may appear unremarkable, even when the disease has extended outside the sinus. Bone erosion is a clear sign that the disease is established, but in general this manifestation is only seen in the later stages of the disease [7, 8]. With aggressive bone destruction, there may be intraorbital and intracranial extension. Vascular infiltration of fungi results in ischemic

Fig. 3 Axial plain CT shows soft tissue in the right maxillary sinus. Note minimal right peri-antral soft tissue thickening (*arrow*), compared to left side clean hypodense peri-antral fat. This was a subtle sign, and biopsy showed invasive mucormycosis

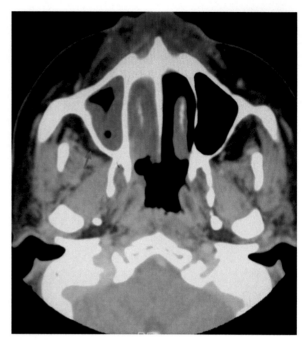

necrosis which results in non-enhancing lesions on post-contrast scans, which are best evaluated on post-gadolinium-enhanced MRI. This also forms the basis of detecting ischemic necrotic areas on perfusion-weighted MR imaging in fungal disease.

It is mandatory to perform detailed MR imaging with multiplanar thin T1- and T2-weighted sections through the skull base, paranasal sinuses, orbits, and any other area clinically indicated, along with post-contrast study, with fat suppression. Additional high-end MRI techniques such as perfusion, diffusion, and MR spectroscopy are now being researched, for better characterization of the disease and its extent. For evaluating intracranial and intraorbital extension of the disease, MRI is superior to CT. On MRI presence of stranding in the orbital fat and swelling with T2 hyperintensity of the extraocular muscles with or without proptosis suggest intraorbital invasion (Figs. 4, 5 and 6).

One of the signs of intracranial extension is leptomeningeal enhancement, which is better appreciated on MRI (Fig. 7). Initially leptomeningeal enhancement may be subtle, and one may really have to look for it [5]. Other findings of intracranial invasion include cerebritis, granulomas, and cerebral abscess formation. A fungal granuloma usually shows hypointense signal on both T1- and T2-weighted images, with minimal enhancement on contrast-enhanced images. At times, intracranial extension may occur directly from the sphenoid sinus into the cavernous sinus. This may lead to cavernous sinus thrombosis and sometimes infiltration into the carotid artery/ occlusion, or pseudoaneurysm, causing ipsilateral large cerebral infarction. Vascular

Fig. 4 MRI coronal post-contrast T1W image shows bilateral ethmoid and maxillary sinus soft tissue, with heterogeneous enhancement. Note ill-defined stranding with enhancement in the superomedial left orbital fat (*small black arrow*), with similar findings around the left optic nerve (*red arrow*), consistent with acute invasive fungal sinusitis

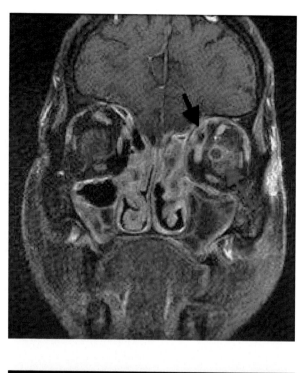

Fig. 5 MRI axial T2W image of the same patient shows bilateral ethmoid opacification, with diffuse fullness and hyperintensity involving the left extraocular muscles (*arrow*), as well as in the retro-ocular fat

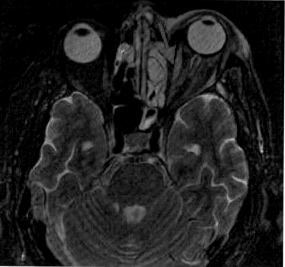

thrombosis is commonly seen with mucormycosis, seen as altered flow signal in a vessel with heterogenous enhancement. This may result in mycotic emboli and cause small abscesses, which are more commonly seen in the frontal lobes.

Fig. 6 MRI T2W coronal image shows predominantly right-sided ethmoid and maxillary mucormycosis, with infiltration into the right orbit (*arrow*)

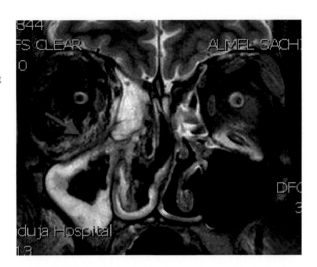

Fig. 7 MRI post-contrast axial T1W image shows intracranial leptomeningeal enhancement in the right frontal region (*arrows*), in the same patient as in Fig. 5, with advanced mucormycosis

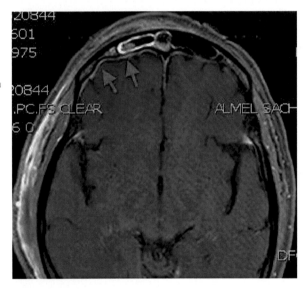

Chronic Invasive Fungal Sinusitis

Fungi, usually, implicated in causing this type of fungal sinusitis are Aspergillus species, dematiaceous molds such as *Bipolaris and Curvularia*, and *Pseudallescheria boydii*. A non-contrast CT may show a hyperattenuating mass-like lesion mimicking a malignancy with destruction of the sinus walls [5] (Fig. 8) and extending beyond the sinus walls into adjacent structures, such as the orbit, maxillary floor/hard palate (Fig. 10 in Chapter "Clinical Features and Diagnosis"), cribriform, or pterygopalatine fossa. The sinus wall may show sclerotic changes on CT suggesting

Fig. 8 Coronal CT scan shows irregular bony destruction of the left maxillary sinus walls (*arrow*) in chronic invasive fungal sinusitis. The patient also had an oroantral fistula, seen at the site of air pocket (*arrow*), along the floor of the left maxillary sinus

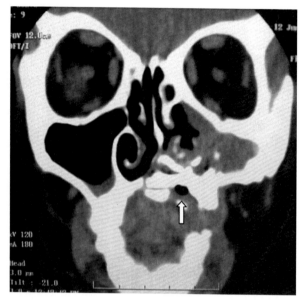

chronicity. There may also be lucencies or irregular bone destruction in the paranasal sinuses. There may also be infiltration of the peri-antral soft tissues around the maxillary sinus. Differentiating malignancy and invasive fungal sinusitis may not be possible on imaging [9, 10]. On MRI, the sinus soft tissue usually shows hypointense signal on both T1 and T2, which at times may be mistaken for air in the sinuses. Presence of iron, magnesium, and increased calcium contents are the causes of T2 shortening. The peri-sinus and intracranial spread is again better evaluated on MRI. Extension of fungal infection intracranially may lead to epidural abscess, parenchymal cerebritis or abscess, meningitis, cavernous sinus thrombosis, osteomyelitis, mycotic aneurysm, stroke, and hematogenous dissemination [5].

Chronic Granulomatous Invasive Sinusitis

This is usually caused by *Aspergillus flavus*. Although there are very few reports describing imaging findings in these patients, cross-sectional imaging findings are expected to be similar to those of chronic invasive fungal sinusitis [5]. Stringer and Ryan [9] have described imaging features similar to those of chronic invasive fungal sinusitis with mass lesion (Fig. 9) in the sinuses eroding the orbital walls and nasal cavity with invasion of the orbital soft tissues and pterygopalatine fossa, difficult to distinguish from a malignant neoplasm.

It is important to be able to compare invasive fungal sinusitis from its noninvasive counterpart, on radiology. Following are the radiological features in noninvasive types of fungal sinus infection.

Fig. 9 CT post-contrast axial image shows hyperdense opacification of the sphenoid sinus, with erosions of its right lateral wall (*arrow*) in a case of chronic granulomatous invasive fungal sinusitis

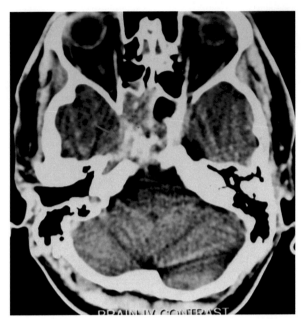

Fig. 10 CT coronal plain image shows large hyperattenuating allergic fungal mass-like lesion in the visualized sphenoid and right maxillary sinus, with expansion of the sphenoid sinus

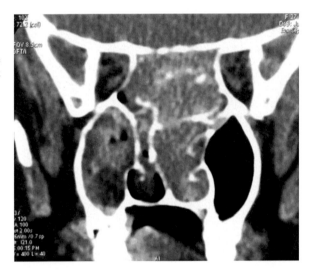

Noninvasive Allergic Fungal Sinusitis

Allergic fungal sinusitis may be bilateral and involves multiple sinuses with near total opacification and expansion of the sinuses. Non-contrast CT scan shows hyperattenuating allergic mucin within the lumen of the paranasal sinus [11] (Figs. 10). This hyperattenuation is due to accumulation of heavy metals (iron, manganese) and calcium salt precipitation within the inspissated allergic fungal mucin. This on MRI

Fig. 11 MRI T2W axial image of another patient with allergic fungal sinusitis shows large T2 hypointense soft tissue (*arrows*), which could almost be mistaken for air

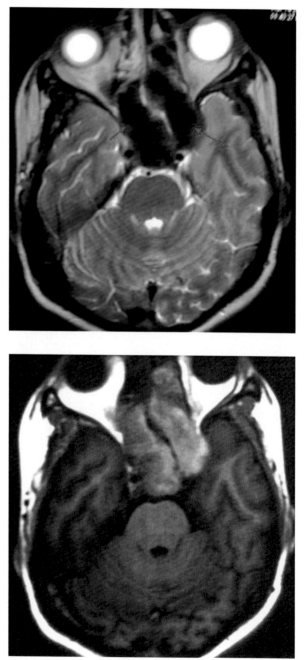

Fig. 12 MRI T1W axial image shows the same soft tissue (as in Fig. 11), to be hyperintense, probably due to proteinaceous contents

(Figs. 11 and 12) is hypointense, on T2W sequences and on T1 may be hyperintense or hypointense. There may be peripheral T2 hyperintense edematous mucosa. Expansion, remodeling, or thinning/erosion of the adjacent bony sinus wall is

Fig. 13 CT coronal image shows a lobulated hyperattenuating fungal ball in the left maxillary sinus

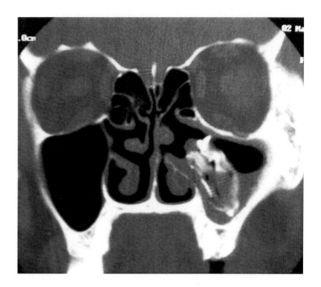

frequently seen, due to the expansile nature of the accumulating mucin. Bony erosions and extension into adjacent vital cavities may be seen in about 20 % cases [11].

Noninvasive Fungal Mycetoma/Ball

A fungal ball or mycetoma affects a single sinus usually the maxillary sinus (Fig. 13) and rarely the sphenoid sinus. The fungal ball appears like a hyperattenuating mass on non-contrast CT scan due to dense matted hyphae. Occasionally there may be punctate calcifications. The bony walls of the sinus may be sclerotic and thickened or expanded and thinned with focal areas of erosion due to pressure necrosis [5]. On MRI, the fungal ball appears hypointense on T1- and T2-weighted images due to the absence of free water. Signal void is also generated on T2-weighted images due to calcifications and paramagnetic metals such as iron, magnesium, and manganese within the mycetoma [5].

References

1. Addlestone RB, Baylin GJ. Rhinocerebral mucormycosis. Radiology. 1975;115:113–7.
2. Green WH, Goldberg HL, Wohl GT. Mucormycosis infection of the craniofacial structures. Am J Roentgenol. 1967;101:802–6.
3. Silverman CS, Mancuso AA. Periantral soft tissue infiltration and its relevance to the early detection of invasive fungal sinusitis: CT and MR findings. AJNR Am J Neuroradiol. 1998;19: 321–5.
4. de Shazo RD, O'Brien M, Chapin K, Soto-Aguilar M, Gardner L, Swain R. A new classification and diagnostic criteria for invasive fungal sinusitis. Arch Otolaryngol. 1997;123:1181–8.

5. Aribandi M, McCoy VA, Bazan C. Imaging features of invasive and non-invasive fungal sinusitis: a review. Radiographics. 2007;27:1283–96.
6. Fatterpekar G, Mukherji S, Arbealez A, Maheshwari S, Castillo M. Fungal diseases of the paranasal sinuses. Semin Ultrasound CT MR. 1999;20(6):391–401.
7. Del Gaudio JM, Clemson LA. An early detection protocol for invasive fungal sinusitis in neutropenic patients successfully reduces extent of disease at presentation and long term morbidity. Laryngoscope. 2009;119:180–3.
8. Gillespie MB, O'Malley BW. Role of middle turbinate biopsy in the diagnosis and management of fulminant invasive fungal rhinosinusitis. Laryngoscope. 2000;110:1832–6.
9. Stringer SP, Ryan MW. Chronic invasive fungal rhinosinusitis. Otolaryngol Clin North Am. 2000;33(2):375–87.
10. Sarti EJ, Blaugrund SM, Lin PT, Camins MB. Paranasal sinus disease with intracranial extension: aspergillosis versus malignancy. Laryngoscope. 1988;98(6 pt 1):632–5.
11. Mukherji SK, Figuerosa RE, Ginsberg LE, et al. Allergic fungal sinusitis: CT findings. Radiology. 1998;207(2):417–22.

Management of Invasive Fungal Sinusitis

Rajeev Soman and Ayesha Sunavala

Introduction

Fungi have long been implicated as important pathogens in selected patients with acute or chronic sinusitis. Inhalation of fungal spores is considered to be the primary means by which these organisms gain access to the sinonasal tract. Fungal sinusitis is an important clinical entity. However, changing terminology and emerging theories of pathogenesis make it an area of confusion and controversy. An analysis of tissue invasion and host immunological response is an important step in the evaluation of the patient.

With intact host defences, infection is usually a benign, non-invasive process restricted to the mucosa. Invasive infections occur typically in immunocompromised hosts and are characterised by fungal proliferation and invasion of vascular structures, leading to thrombosis of vessels with resultant tissue necrosis. Eventually, the fungi extend beyond the affected sinus via bony destruction, perineural and perivascular spread. The most common fungi involved are Aspergillus species and the Mucorales. Less common causative agents are Candida, Pseudallescheria, Fusarium and the dematiaceous fungi [1].

The management of these invasive fungal infections (Fig. 1) is fraught with myriad challenges. The choice of the empirical antifungal agent based on host factors and clinical and radiological findings is extremely difficult as the triazoles, with the exception of posaconazole, are ineffective for mucormycosis. Secondly, based on the severity and duration of the immunosuppressive condition, invasive fungal infections may follow a fulminant, often fatal course requiring emergent therapeutic intervention. This involves rapid reversal of causative host factors, immediate surgical debridement if possible and the careful administration of antifungals with

R. Soman, MD (✉) • A. Sunavala, DNB
Department of Internal Medicine and Infectious Diseases,
PD Hinduja Hospital, Mahim, Mumbai, Maharashtra, India
e-mail: rajeev.soman@yahoo.com

G. Mankekar (ed.), *Invasive Fungal Rhinosinusitis*,
DOI 10.1007/978-81-322-1530-1_8, © Springer India 2014

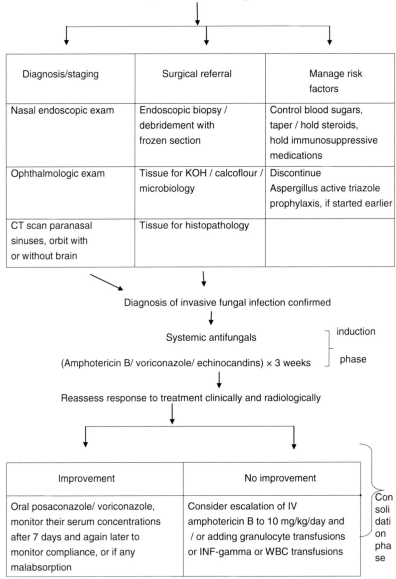

Fig. 1 Management of patient with IFS

close monitoring of their toxicities and drug interactions. Finally, the response and duration of therapy is based on the judgement of the treating physician and may be especially challenging in chronically immunosuppressed patients.

As the choice of treatment for mucormycosis is so different from that of other moulds, it is important to bear in mind factors pointing to mucormycosis.

Factors Favouring Mucormycosis Over Aspergillosis [2]

Epidemiological and host clues:

1. Institution with high background rates of mucormycosis
2. Iron overload states
3. Hyperglycemia with/without DM
4. Prior voriconazole or echinocandin use

Clinical, radiological and laboratory clues:

1. Community-acquired sinusitis
2. Oral necrotic lesions on the hard palate or nasal turbinates
3. Serosanguineous bloodstained or dark nasal discharge
4. Repeatedly negative serum galactomannan

Management of Invasive Mucormycosis

Correction of Predisposing Factors

Tapering of immunosuppressive therapy may not be feasible especially in transplant recipients. However, tapering or discontinuation of corticosteroids is advised with the added benefit of better glycaemic control and reduced risk of ketoacidosis.

Diabetic ketoacidosis increases the availability of free iron available to Mucorales and is the most frequent underlying risk factor for mucormycosis in the developing world. Hyperglycaemia associated with long-term high-dose corticosteroid therapy is a key 'late' risk factor for breakthrough mucormycosis, although it is unknown whether tighter glycaemic control reduces this risk [2].

Neutropenia should be rapidly corrected by initiation of granulocyte colony-stimulating factors (G-CSF) as well as discontinuation of chemotherapeutic agents responsible for marrow suppression [3].

Surgical Debridement

Early, aggressive and repeated surgical excision of necrotic craniofacial tissues is the cornerstone of successful management. This in conjunction with systemic antifungals has shown significant survival benefit. This may be explained by the fact that angioinvasion, thrombosis and tissue necrosis associated with mucormycosis lead to poor penetration of antifungal agents at the sites of infection and compromise their efficacy [4]. Small focal lesions should be surgically resected without delay before they progress to involve critical structures or distal organs. The limits of debridement can be decided by the use of intraoperative frozen sections, also known as the 'conservative-aggressive approach' [5]. Repeated removal of necrotic tissue, extensive, disfiguring debridement of the sinuses and enucleation of orbit may be required to prevent dissemination to critical structures. Decisions about the timing and extent of debridement are often made at the bedside [2]. Subsequent plastic surgery may also be in order to cosmetically address anatomic defects.

Systemic Antifungal Agents (Table 1)

Polyenes are currently the preferred therapeutic agents for mucormycosis.

Several studies suggest that lipid formulations of amphotericin B, particularly liposomal amphotericin B (LAmB), are associated with improved response rates (partial and complete) or survival. In patients receiving amphotericin B deoxycholate (AmBD) as primary therapy, combined complete and partial response rates range from 0 to 60 %, and all-cause mortality varies from 39 to 75 %. Whereas, in patients receiving LAmB as primary or salvage therapy, combined complete and partial response rates are 32–100 %, and overall mortality ranges from 5 to 61 % [5].

The lipid formulations offer a definite advantage as compared to AmBD for transplant recipients due to fewer nephrotoxic effects, for central nervous system infections as they have superior brain penetration, but they are expensive. In addition to improved CNS penetration, LAmB may be advantageous to the host as it possesses unique immunomodulatory characteristics, thus, lowering the risk of inflammatory tissue pathology, whereas AmBD has pro-inflammatory properties, leading to increased cytokine production and tissue destruction [6].

Posaconazole is the only FDA approved azole with in vitro activity against the Mucorales. However, pharmacokinetic-pharmacodynamic (PKPD) data raise concerns about the reliability of achieving adequate in vivo levels with orally administered posaconazole [7]. Secondly, posaconazole is found to be inferior to AmB for the treatment of murine mucormycosis especially in neutropenics. Thus, posaconazole is not recommended as a primary therapy for mucormycosis. Furthermore, combined posaconazole and AmBD or LAmB offered no survival benefit over AmBD or LAmB alone [5].

Patients who respond to a parenteral AmB-based treatment, given for at least 3 weeks, may then be transitioned over several days, to oral posaconazole as maintenance/secondary prophylaxis, as the steady-state plasma concentration of posaconazole is not achieved until 1 week of therapy [3]. It is common for patients especially those with haematologic malignancies, chemotherapy-induced mucositis, diarrhoea or graft-versus-host disease (GVHD) to have multiple risk factors for malabsorption, frequently leading to undetectable serum concentrations of posaconazole and hence breakthrough infections. In addition, posaconazole is also a potent inhibitor of CYP enzymes, leading to numerous and often unpredictable drug interactions especially with other immunosuppressive agents. Therefore, current strategies to

Table 1 Antifungal agents for mucormycosis

Drug	Dose	Advantages	Disadvantages	Special precautions
AmBD	1–1.5 mg/kg/day	Inexpensive Maximum experience	Nephrotoxicity Poor CNS penetration	Test dose, premedication to prevent hypersensitivity reaction
LAmB	5–10 mg/kg/day	Less nephrotoxicity Good CNS penetration	Expensive	
Amphotericin B lipid complex (ABLC)	5–7.5 mg/kg/day	Less nephrotoxicity Clinical studies suggest benefit with combination therapy with echinocandins	Expensive Less efficacious than LAmB for CNS infections	
Caspofungin plus lipid polyene	70-mg IV loading dose, then 50 mg/day for 2 weeks	Favourable toxicity profile Synergistic in murine dissemi-nated mucormycosis Retrospective clinical data suggest superior outcomes for rhino-orbital-cerebral mucormycosis	Limited data on combination therapy Limited penetration into CNS	
Posaconazole	800 mg/day PO in 4 divided doses	Oral administration for salvage, maintenance/ secondary prophylaxis	Uncertain bioavailability Requires drug level monitoring Breakthrough infections reported, not to be used as primary treatment 7 days to reach steady-state concentration	Must be co-administered with fatty foods, acidic beverages Avoid proton pump inhibitors

Adapted from Spellberg and Ibrahim [7]

improve posaconazole serum concentrations are focused primarily on improving drug dissolution and absorption (i.e. administer with high-fat food, acidic beverage), discontinuing acid suppression therapy (especially proton pump inhibitors) and regular serum drug level monitoring [2].

The new triazole isavuconazole, currently undergoing clinical trials, is found to be active against moulds including Mucormycotina [8].

Although the echinocandins are deemed inactive against Glomeromycota, small studies have shown improved response rates of combination therapy with LAmB and caspofungin. Whether the observed survival benefits result from the effect of combination therapy on improved polyene delivery to the cell membrane after disruption of β-glucan in the cell wall or are due to immunomodulation of the host response remains to be determined [5].

The duration of therapy is highly individualised and should be decided based upon recovery from immunosuppression or reversal of other contributing host factors, improvement in radiological imaging and negative biopsy specimens/cultures from repeated debridement of the affected site [3].

Adjunctive Treatments

1. Hyperbaric oxygen therapy has been found to be a beneficial adjunctive therapy for mucormycosis, particularly diabetic patients with rhinocerebral disease [9]. Specifically, the increased partial pressure of oxygen achieved with hyperbaric therapy seems to improve neutrophil activity and oxidative killing by amphotericin B. In addition, high concentrations of oxygen can inhibit the growth of Mucorales in vitro and improve the rate of wound healing by increasing the release of tissue growth factors [10]. There are no clinical data to suggest appropriate pressures and duration of therapy. It is usually started during the acute phase of the illness and not as salvage therapy at 2.4–3.0 ATA range of pressures, twice daily depending on the patient's general condition and ability to tolerate the pressures. In some successful cases up to 30 treatments have been reported [11].
2. Iron plays a pivotal role in the pathogenesis of mucormycosis, its proliferative and angioinvasive properties. The role of deferasirox, an iron chelator without xenosiderophore activity in Mucorales, was emphasised in a recent case series from our centre. Deferasirox starves the fungus of iron which is critical for its growth and pathogenicity [12].
3. Immune augmentation strategies are also considered in patients with refractory mucormycosis, including administration of cytokines (e.g. granulocyte-macrophage colony-stimulating factor, interferon). In select neutropenic patients, granulocyte transfusion may be a useful bridge until neutrophil recovery, although the clinical benefit remains unproven; and serious adverse effects, including pulmonary toxicity and accelerated cavitation/bleeding, have been reported in patients with opportunistic lung mycoses [5].

4. Research reveals that both yeast and moulds have homologues of calcineurin and mTOR that play a significant part in fungal growth and proliferation. Hence, in addition to their immunosuppressive effects, the calcineurin inhibitors (tacrolimus, cyclosporin) and mTOR inhibitors (sirolimus, everolimus) have been found to have antifungal activity against both yeast and moulds [5]. The potential clinical relevance of this development needs to be further explored as knowledge of interactions between antifungal agents and immunosuppressants could improve outcomes.

5. Another potential adjunctive agent currently under study is colistin which has been shown to exert fungicidal activity in vitro against *R. oryzae* by damaging cytoplasmic and vacuolar membranes, leading to the leakage of intracellular contents [13].

6. Statins have been found to have fungicidal activity against Glomeromycota and act synergistically with other antifungal agents, such as voriconazole [14].

Management of Invasive Sinonasal Aspergillosis

Several studies involving immunocompromised patients indicate that sinonasal aspergillosis may be associated with invasive pulmonary aspergillosis or complicated by CNS or orbital invasion [15]. Despite appropriate host factors and strong clinical suspicion of possible aspergillosis, if the identification of the aetiological organism is unknown or pending, an AmB formulation should be initiated to also cover possible mucormycosis. When the diagnosis of confirmed or probable invasive aspergillosis has been established, voriconazole is considered to be the drug of choice. AmBD has also been approved for primary treatment; however, due to high rates of nephrotoxicity and excess mortality attributed to it, use of lipid formulations or alternative agents is preferred. Lipid formulations of AmB, itraconazole, posaconazole and caspofungin are advocated as salvage therapy for patients who are refractory to or intolerant of primary therapy [16, 17]. Posaconazole has been approved in the European Union for treatment of invasive aspergillosis that is refractory to an AmB formulation or to itraconazole. Micafungin and anidulafungin have shown in vitro, in vivo and clinical activity against aspergillosis but are not licensed in the USA for this indication as yet [17]. Posaconazole has also been licensed for use as prophylaxis in neutropenic patients with haematological malignancies and in allogenic haematopoietic stem cell transplant (HSCT) patients with graft-versus-host disease GVHD [16]. Table 2 shows the indications, doses and characteristics of anti-fungal agents used in the treatment of invasive aspergillosis.

The duration of therapy for invasive aspergillosis has not been clearly defined and may have to be continued for at least 3 months. Most experts prefer to continue treatment until resolution or stabilisation of all clinical and radiographic manifestations. Other factors involved in deciding treatment duration include

Table 2 Indications, doses and characteristics of antifungal agents in the management of invasive aspergillosis [17]

Drug	Dosage	Indication	Advantages	Disadvantages
Voriconazole	6 mg/kg IV 12hrly on day1, followed by 4 mg/kg 12hrly	Primary therapy	Oral formulation may be used as step down therapy after initial stabilisation with IV preparation	IV formulation not to be used if GFR <50. (Oral formulation may be used)
	6 mg/kg 12hrly on day1 followed by 3 mg/kg 12hrly (Oral dose 200 mg BID)	Empirical and pre-emptive therapy		CYP2C19 substrate and inducer with multiple, significant drug interactions
				Monitoring of drug levels required
LAmB	3–5 mg/kg/day IV	Alternative/salvage therapy	No nephrotoxicity	Optimal dose for invasive aspergillosis not defined
	3 mg/kg/day IV	Empirical and pre-emptive therapy	Reduced hypersensitivity reactions	Inactive against A. terreus, A. nidulans
ABLC	5 mg/kg/day IV	Same as above		
Caspofungin	70 mg IV OD on day 1, followed by 50 mg IV OD	Alternative/salvage therapy	No renal dose adjustment required	Drug interactions with calcineurin inhibitors (immunosuppressants), antiretrovirals, rifampicin, antiepileptics, dexamethasone
		Empirical and pre-emptive therapy		Dose reduction in hepatic dysfunction
Posaconazole	200 mg PO QID until disease stabilisation followed by 400 mg BID	Alternative/salvage therapy	Oral formulation	Steady-state level not achieved for 1 week. (Not to be used as primary therapy)
	200 mg PO TID	Prophylaxis against invasive pulmonary aspergillosis		Must be co-administered with fatty foods, acidic beverages. Avoid proton pump inhibitors

Itraconazole	600 mg/day PO × 3 days followed by 400 mg/day PO	Alternative/salvage therapy	Oral formulation	Not recommended in critical patient/life-threatening infection due to erratic absorption (improved with acidic foods)
	200 mg PO BID	Empirical and pre-emptive therapy		Negative inotrope; caution in pts. with ventricular dysfunction
		Alternative agent for prophylaxis of invasive pulmonary aspergillosis		Drug interactions with certain chemotherapeutic agents
				Monitoring of drug levels advised

the site of infection, level of ongoing immunosuppression and extent of disease.

A growing body of evidence suggests patient-to-patient variability in the pharmacokinetics of triazoles used for treatment or prophylaxis in invasive aspergillosis. Absorption issues (for itraconazole and posaconazole), drug-drug interactions (for all triazoles) and pharmacogenetic differences (for voriconazole) all contribute in various degrees to this variability, and hence plasma drug level monitoring may play an important role in optimising the safety and efficacy of the triazole antifungals [17].

Voriconazole is extensively metabolised in the liver by CYP2C19 drug-metabolising enzyme. This enzyme has various genetic polymorphisms which affect the rate of drug metabolism, leading to a considerable impact on the dose of drug required to achieve therapeutic plasma levels [17]. Studies reveal that 12–14 % of Indians have CYP2 C19 polymorphisms [18], and hence it may be prudent to check for these mutations especially in critical patients where attaining therapeutic drug levels may significantly affect outcome.

Surgical Management

Surgical evaluation should be conducted urgently for both diagnostic biopsy and debridement [19]. This is difficult in some patients because of the extent of the infection or the severity of the underlying disease. However, invasive sinus aspergillosis may be complicated by cavernous sinus thrombosis or invasion into critical structures of the CNS and orbit, hence, prompt surgical debridement of involved tissues plays an important role in management and may even be curative in some circumstances. Local irrigation with AmB is sometimes administered by the surgical team as an adjunct to systemic antifungals post debridement. However, it is difficult to assess objectively the efficacy of this line of treatment as surgery alone may be curative [20].

Adjunctive Measures

The vital role of reduction or discontinuation of immunosuppression in successful outcome cannot be overemphasised. However, this may not always be achievable. Neutropenic patients may benefit significantly from the addition of colony-stimulating factors (G-CSF, GM-CSF). Individual case reports suggest the role of IFN-γ as an adjunct to augment phagocytic function [17].

Management of Other Fungi Causing Invasive Fungal Sinusitis (Table 3) [19, 21]

Table 3 Enumerates the antifungal agents used to manage patients with invasive fungal sinusitis due to other fungi

	Primary treatment	Alternative treatment	Duration	Intrinsic resistance
Fusarium	Voriconazole	LAmB, AmBD, posaconazole	Prolonged, at least 6 months after recovery from neutropenia	Fluconazole, itraconazole, 5 flucyto-sine, caspofungin
Pseudallescheria boydii/ Scedosporium apiospermum	Voriconazole	Posaconazole- not licensed (good in vitro activity)	6–12 months guided by clinical resolution	85 % isolates resistant to AmB
Dematiaceous fungi	AmB + azole in combination (voriconazole/ itraconazole/ posaconazole)	Polyene or azole alone	At least 6 months, may be longer up to 2 years	

Table 3 enumerates the antifungal agents used to manage patients with invasive fungal sinusitis due to other fungi. Effective management of invasive fungal sinusitis requires a team approach involving surgeons, histopathologists, microbiologists and physicians. Reversal of the underlying predisposition, surgery, antifungal treatment, adjunctive therapy and close follow-up remain important components of management.

Duration of Treatment

As far as possible, the treatment of invasive fungal sinusitis should be highly individualised and continued until there is clinical resolution of all symptoms and signs [2]. Follow-up cultures should be negative with reversal of underlying metabolic derangements or immunosuppression. Serial imaging should have resolution of radiographic signs of active disease with the exception of radiologic findings thought to be the result of inflammation or surgery. Chamilos et al. [22] have suggested that positron emission CT may be useful in making this distinction in some patients. In view of late recurrences, especially of mucormycosis, in patients who have been previously treated successfully but required subsequent chemotherapy, Kontoyiannis et al. do not recommend discontinuation of antifungals early [2].

Monitoring of Relapse

No biomarkers or approaches have been identified to monitor relapse of invasive fungal sinusitis. Intensification of immunosuppression, metabolic derangement (e.g. uncontrolled hyperglycaemia), relapse of leukaemia, cytomegalovirus reactivation, drug-related issues (non-compliance, drug interactions) and the presence of anatomic sequestra are factors that increase the risk of recurrent infection [2]. Patients should be followed up at regular intervals with appropriate cultures and biopsies. Moussett et al. [23] tried white blood cell transfusion as secondary prophylaxis in a small series of high-risk patients with severe fungal infection who were at risk of relapse of their mycoses.

Prognosis

The mortality rates for invasive fungal infections, especially mucormycosis, exceed 60 % [24]. Prognosis is determined by the site of infection and underlying host factors, especially, the underlying status of haematologic disease and immunosuppression [25, 26]. Pagano et al. [26] reported that in a series of 391 patients with haematologic malignancies, most patients who developed mucormycosis died within 12 weeks of diagnosis compared to patients with aspergillosis who had a significantly better prognosis. Also, some unusual Mucorales like *Cunninghamella* spp. are associated with poor overall prognosis compared to the more common Rhizopus species, probably due to the inherently greater resistance of *Cunninghamella* species to antifungal agents and polymorphonuclear leukocyte-mediated hyphal damage [27].

References

1. Demuri GP, Wald ER. Sinusitis. In: Mandell GL, Benett JE, Dolin R, editors. Principles and practice of infectious diseases, vol. 2. 7th ed. Philadelphia: Elsevier Churchill Livingstone; 2010. p. 842.
2. Kontoyiannis DP, Lewis RE. How I treat mucormycosis. Blood. 2011;118(5):1216–24.
3. Kontoyiannis DP, Lewis RE. Agents of mucormycosis and entomophthoromycosis. In: Mandell GL, Bennett JE, Dolin R, editors. Principles and practice of infectious diseases, vol. 2. 7th ed. Philadelphia: Elsevier Churchill Livingstone; 2010. p. 3257–67.
4. Spellberg B, Edwards Jr J, Ibrahim A. Novel perspectives on mucormycosis: pathophysiology, presentation, and management. Clin Microbiol Rev. 2005;18:556–69.
5. Sun HY, Singh N. Mucormycosis: its contemporary face and management strategies. Lancet Infect Dis. 2011;11(4):301–11.
6. Ben-Ami R, Lewis RE, Kontoyiannis DP. Immunocompromised hosts: immunopharmacology of modern antifungals. Clin Infect Dis. 2008;47:226–35.
7. Spellberg B, Ibrahim AS, et al. Mucormycosis. In: Longo DL, editor. Harrison's principles of internal medicine. 18th ed. London: The McGraw-Hill Companies, Inc.; 2012. p. 1663–6.

8. Thompson 3rd GR, Wiederhold NP. Isavuconazole: a comprehensive review of spectrum of activity of a new triazole. Mycopathologia. 2010;170:291–313.
9. John BV, Chamilos G, Kontoyiannis DP. Hyperbaric oxygen as an adjunctive treatment for zygomycosis. Clin Microbiol Infect. 2005;11(7):515–7.
10. Kaide CG, Khandelwal S. Hyperbaric oxygen: applications in infectious disease. Emerg Med Clin North Am. 2008;26(2):571–95.
11. Neuman TS, Thom SR, editors. Physiology and rationale of hyperbaric oxygen therapy. Philadelphia: Saunders Elsevier; 2008. pp 321–47.
12. Soman R, Gupta N, Shetty A, Rodrigues C. Deferasirox in mucormycosis: hopefully, not defeated. J Antimicrob Chemother. 2012;67(3):783–4.
13. Ben-Ami R, Lewis RE, Tarrand J, Leventakos K, Kontoyiannis DP. Antifungal activity of colistin against mucorales species in vitro and in a murine model of Rhizopus oryzae pulmonary infection. Antimicrob Agents Chemother. 2010;54:484–90.
14. Terblanche M, Almog Y, Rosenson RS, Smith TS, Hackam DG. Statins and sepsis: multiple modifications at multiple levels. Lancet Infect Dis. 2007; 7:358–68.
15. Ashdown B, Tien R, Felsberg G. Aspergillosis of the brain and paranasal sinuses in immunocompromised patients: CT and MR imaging findings. AJR Am J Roentgenol. 1994;162: 155–9.
16. Patterson TF. Aspergillus species. In: Mandell GL, Benett JE, Dolin R, editors. Principles and practice of infectious diseases, vol. 2. 7th ed. Philadelphia: Elsevier Churchill Livingstone; 2010. p. 3241–55.
17. Walsh TJ, Anaissie EJ, Denning DW, et al. Treatment of aspergillosis: clinical practice guidelines of the infectious diseases society of America. Clin Infect Dis. 2008;46:327–60.
18. Chaudhary AS, Kochhar R, Kohli KK. Genetic polymorphism of CYP2C19 & therapeutic response to proton pump inhibitors. Indian J Med Res. 2008;127:521–30.
19. Cox GM, Perfect JR. Fungal rhinosinusitis. [homepage on the Internet]. 2012 [cited 25 Feb 2013]. Available from: http://www.uptodate.com.
20. De Carpentier JE, Ramamurthy L, Denning DW, Taylor PH. An algorithmic approach to aspergillus sinusitis. J Laryngol Otol. 1994;108:314–8.
21. Zaas A. Fusarium, Scedosporium [homepage on the internet]. 2012 [cited 25 Feb 2013]. Available from: http://www.hopkinsguides.com.
22. Chamilos G, Macapinlac HA, Kontoyiannis DP. The use of 18F-fluorodeoxyglucose positron emission tomography for the diagnosis and management of invasive mold infections. Med Mycol. 2008;46(1):23–9.
23. Moussett S, Hermann S, Klein SA, et al. Prophylactic and interventional granulocyte transfusions in patients with haematological malignancies and life-threatening infections during neutropenia. Ann Hematol. 2005;84(11):734–41.
24. Herbrecht R, Letscher-Bru V, Bowden RA, et al. Treatment of 21 cases of invasive mucormycosis with amphotericin B colloidal dispersion. Eur J Clin Microbiol Infect Dis. 2001;20: 460–6.
25. Chamilos G, Lewis RE, Kontoyiannis DP. Delaying Amphotericin B- based frontline therapy significantly increases mortality among patients with hematologic malignancy who have zygomycosis. Clin Infect Dis. 2008;47(4):503–9.
26. Pagano L, Akova M, Dimopoulos G, et al. Risk assessment and prognostic factors for mold related diseases in immunocompromised patients. J Antimicrob Chemother. 2011;66(1): i5–14.
27. Gomes MZ, Lewis RE, Kontoyiannis DP. Mucormycosis caused by unusual mucormycetes, non-rhizopus, mucor and lichtheimia species. Clin Microbiol Rev. 2011;24(2):411–45.

Conclusion

Gauri Mankekar

Differentiating between the types of fungal sinusitis and identifying the aggressive fulminant type are crucial to the management of patients of invasive fungal sinusitis (Table 1). In order to improve outcomes of invasive fungal sinusitis, several factors require to be addressed. Education and training of medical personnel to identify the disease early forms the crux of successful management along with meticulous infection control practices, policies to control infection during construction and renovation of hospitals and early recognition of nosocomial outbreaks. Additionally concomitant research to understand the immunopathogenesis of the disease, immunogenetic risk factors for invasive fungal infections in humans and the development of diagnostic (such as PCR techniques and biomarkers) as well as therapeutic modalities (like immunopharmacology and vaccines) can improve outcomes. With the development of genome sequencing and molecular tools for studying fungi, this may all be soon possible.

G. Mankekar, MS, DNB, PhD
ENT, PD Hinduja Hospital, Mahim, Mumbai,
Maharashtra 400 016, India
e-mail: gaurimankekar@gmail.com

G. Mankekar (ed.), *Invasive Fungal Rhinosinusitis*,
DOI 10.1007/978-81-322-1530-1_9, © Springer India 2014

Table 1 Comparative features of fungal sinusitis

Syndrome	Fungi	Geographic distribution	Host factor	Associated conditions	Histopathology	Clinical features	Treatment	Prognosis
Acute fulminant invasive fungal sinusitis	Fungi of the order Mucorales and *Aspergillus fumigatus*	Worldwide	Immunocompromised but also seen in immune competent	Diabetes, hematologic malignancies, steroid therapy, immunosuppressive therapy, organ transplants	Sparse fungal elements in mucosa, submucosa, blood vessels, bone, with extensive tissue necrosis and neutrophilic inflammation	Chronic sinusitis, proptosis, orbital chemosis	Debridement, systemic antifungals, management of underlying metabolic conditions and immune suppression	High rate of morbidity and mortality
Chronic invasive	*Aspergillus fumigatus or Mucorales*	No specific geographic location	Immunocompromised	Diabetes mellitus	Dense accumulation of fungal elements in a mucoid matrix forming an expansile mass with low-grade chronic inflammatory response in adjacent mucosa	Rhinosinusitis (often unilateral), nasal obstruction, green brown nasal discharge, with or without bone necrosis and sequestrum	Debridement, aeration Antifungals not required	Excellent
Granulomatous invasive	*Aspergillus flavus*	Predominantly reported from Sudan	Immunocompetent	None	Fungal elements in mucosa, submucosa, blood vessels or bone with extensive tissue necrosis and neutrophilic inflammation	Nasal block, nasal crusting, epistaxis, cheek swelling or proptosis with diplopia	Radical debridement, antifungal antibiotic	Fair when limited to sinus; could be variable with intracranial involve-ment

Allergic fungal sinusitis	*Bipolaris spicifera* or *Curvularia lunata* or *Aspergillus* species like *A. fumigatus*, *A. flavus* or *A. niger*	Worldwide	Immuno-competent	None or allergies	Allergic mucin with Charcot-Leyden crystals with absence of tissue invasion	Chronic pansinusitis with nasal polyps, mucus with consistency of "peanut butter"	Debridement, aeration, oral and topical steroids, immuno-therapy. Itraconazole may reduce incidence of recurrence	Recurrence common
Fungal ball or myce-toma	*Aspergillus* spp.	Worldwide	Immuno-competent	None	Compactly packed septate branching fungal hyphae, morphologically resembling *Aspergillus* spp.	Foul smelling nasal discharge, usually single sinus involvement with calcification within the sinus seen on CT	Debridement, aeration. No antifungals	Good

Adapted from DeShazo [1–3]

References

1. de Shazo RD. Syndromes of invasive fungal sinusitis. Med Mycol. 2009;47(Suppl I): S309–14.
2. de Shazo RD, Swain RE. Diagnostic criteria for allergic fungal sinusitis. J Allergy Clin Immunol. 1995;96:24–35.
3. de Shazo RD, O'Brien M, Chapin K, et al. Criteria for the diagnosis of sinus mycetoma. J Allergy Clin Immunol. 1997;99:475–85.

Case Studies

Gauri Mankekar

Several cases can mimic invasive fungal rhinosinusitis, either clinically or radiologically or both. This causes confusion and controversy among clinicians with misdirection of treatment. A few such cases are discussed here.

Case 1

A 26-year-old immunocompetent lady came with complaints of recurrent rhinitis, headaches, and right diplopia since 4 days. On nasal endoscopy, there was grossly deviated septum to the right with multiple polyps (arrow) in the left nasal cavity (Fig. 1). CT scan of paranasal sinuses was obtained (Figs. 2 and 3).

The patient underwent endoscopic nasal clearance of the sinuses. Intraoperatively, there was inspissated pus and debris (arrow) (Fig. 4) in both the sphenoid sinuses, but the lining mucosa of the sinuses appeared normal.

Histopathology showed typical features of allergic fungal sinusitis (Fig. 4).

The patient was started on oral and topical nasal steroids with nasal douching following surgery. Three months postoperatively, the patient's diplopia recovered and the appearance of the sphenoid sinus is shown in Fig. 5.

Discussion: Allergic fungal sinusitis (AFS) is a noninvasive form of fungal rhinosinusitis. It contributes to approximately 6–9 % of all rhinosinusitis requiring surgery [1]. Patients of AFS usually present with chronic rhinosinusitis with nasal polyps, atopy, and elevated total serum IgE, and their sinuses are filled with characteristic "peanut butter"-like eosinophil-rich "allergic mucin" containing sparse fungal hyphae. CT scan of the sinuses (Figs. 2 and 3) is always abnormal, usually showing bilateral and multiple sinus involvement with near total opacification and

G. Mankekar, MS, DNB, PhD
ENT, PD Hinduja Hospital, Mahim, Mumbai,
Maharashtra 400 016, India
e-mail: gaurimankekar@gmail.com

G. Mankekar (ed.), *Invasive Fungal Rhinosinusitis*,
DOI 10.1007/978-81-322-1530-1_10, © Springer India 2014

Fig. 1 Nasal endoscopy
showing left nasal polyposis
with allergic "peanut butter"
mucin (*arrow*)

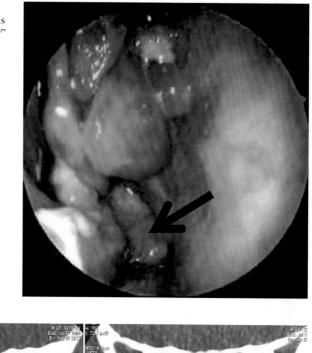

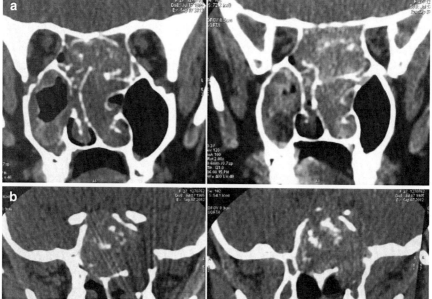

Fig. 2 (**a, b**) Case 1: Coronal plain CT scan (soft tissue settings) showing extensive polypoid soft tissue in both ethmoid, sphenoid, and right maxillary sinuses. Note irregular hyperdense areas within them, which may be due to inspissation or superadded fungal infection

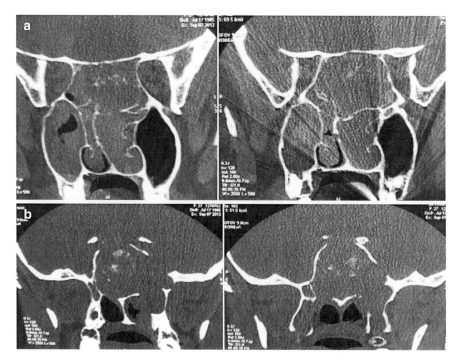

Fig. 3 (**a, b**) Case 1: Coronal plain CT scan (bone window settings) showing marked attenuation of the bony ethmoid wall, with erosions in the sphenoid sinus wall. Note extension of soft tissue inferiorly towards the left pterygoid and left lateral parasphenoid regions

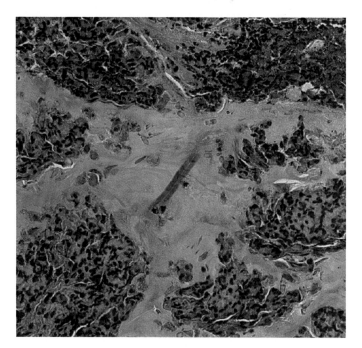

Fig. 4 H&E stain showing allergic fungal mucin with Charcot-Leyden crystals

Fig. 5 Case 1: 6 weeks
post-op endoscopic
appearance of the right
sphenoid sinus

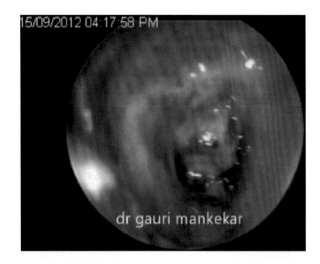

expansion of the sinuses. Expansion, remodeling, or thinning/erosion of the adjacent bony sinus wall is frequently seen, due to the expansile nature of the accumulating mucin. Bony erosions and extension into adjacent vital cavities may be seen in about 20 % cases [1]. AFS allergic mucin, on culture, is typically positive for either dematiaceous fungi like *Bipolaris spicifera* or *Curvularia lunata* or *Aspergillus* species like *A. fumigatus*, *A. flavus*, or *A. niger* [2]. Cases of allergic fungal sinusitis with loss of bony architecture on imaging studies may be misinterpreted as evidence of bony invasion [3] and labeled as invasive fungal sinusitis. But histopathology showing absence of tissue invasion should enable the clinician to diagnose AFS and differentiate it from other forms of both noninvasive and invasive fungal sinusitis. The patient of AFS can be managed with surgical debridement, systemic and local steroids, and nasal douching without systemic antifungals.

Patients with allergic fungal sinusitis showing tissue invasion on histopathology are being encountered and are being termed as "mixed" infection. Such a progression may be due to change in host defenses [4]. These cases may require systemic antifungals, in addition to surgical debridement, nasal douching, and regular follow-up with nasal endoscopy and radiological imaging. Reports suggest oral itraconazole therapy, especially in recalcitrant cases, may avoid or delay revision surgery [5, 6] and even enable patients to reduce or even stop oral steroid therapy [6].

Case 2

A 55-year-old male patient came with history of foul smelling breath with left purulent rhinorrhea. On examination, his left nasal cavity showed purulent discharge from the left middle meatus region (Fig. 6). A CT scan of the paranasal sinuses was done (Fig. 7).

Fig. 6 Endoscopic picture of foul smelling purulent discharge from the left middle meatus

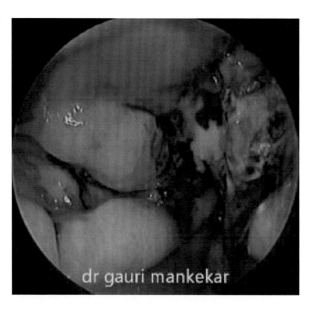

Fig. 7 Case 2: CT coronal image shows a lobulated hyperattenuating fungal ball in the left maxillary sinus

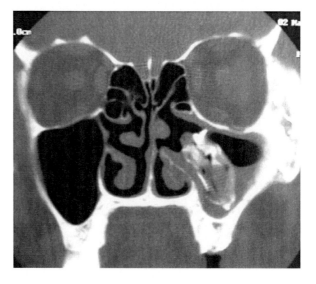

The patient underwent endoscopic debridement of the left maxillary sinus. Intra-op endoscopic appearance of the fungal ball is shown in Fig. 8.

Histopathological appearance is shown in Fig. 9.

Subsequently he was started on saline nasal douches and completely recovered.

Discussion: A fungal ball or mycetoma or aspergilloma or chronic noninvasive granuloma is described as the presence of noninvasive accumulation of dense conglomeration of fungal hyphae in one sinus cavity. It usually affects a single sinus,

Fig. 8 Intra-op endoscopic appearance of the fungal ball (*arrow*)

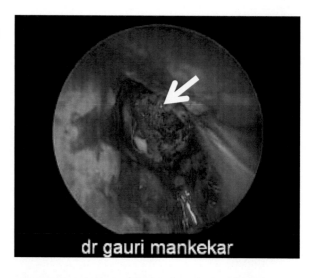

dr gauri mankekar

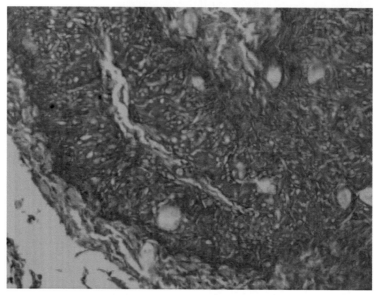

Fig. 9 Histopathology: H&E stain (original magnification 400×) showing fungal ball with compactly packed septate branching fungal hyphae, morphologically resembling *Aspergillus* spp

commonly the maxillary sinus and rarely the sphenoid sinus [7]. It is more common in middle-aged and elderly females, in contrast to invasive sinusitis and aspergillosis which are common in males [8]. The disease is identified due to its characteristic radiologic appearance (Fig. 7) – single sinus opacification with or without radiographic heterogeneity; mucopurulent, cheesy, or clay-like material within the sinus, a dense conglomeration of hyphae separate from the sinus mucosa; nonspecific

Fig. 10 Case 3: Coronal plain CT scan (soft tissue settings) shows polypoidal soft tissue in the right maxillary sinus, with linear hyperdensity within it

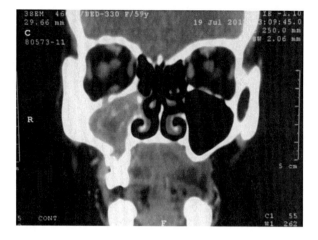

chronic inflammation of the mucosa; lack of predominance of eosinophils or granuloma or allergic mucin; and lack of evidence of mucosal invasion on histopathology [9]. The fungal ball appears like a hyperattenuating mass on non-contrast CT scan due to dense matted hyphae. Occasionally there may be punctate calcifications. The bony walls of the sinus may be sclerotic and thickened or expanded and thinned with focal areas of erosion due to pressure necrosis. On MRI, the fungal ball appears hypointense on T1- and T2-weighted images due to the absence of free water. Signal void is also generated on T2-weighted images due to calcifications and paramagnetic metals such as iron, magnesium, and manganese within the mycetoma.

Such cases could be clinically and radiologically mistaken as invasive fungal sinusitis. But histopathology is diagnostic (Fig. 9) as it does not show tissue invasion. The fungi remain noninvasive in the context of the fungal ball, but could rarely become invasive after substantial immunosuppression, such as in renal transplantation [10]. Identification of Aspergillus species as the causative agent may be aided by the use of galactomannan detection in the sinus material [11].

Surgical debridement, as in this patient, is the only treatment required.

Case 3

A 59-year-old lady came with complaints of severe pain along the right cheek with diplopia and photophobia. She had history of recurrent rhinitis and had undergone a CT scan of the paranasal sinuses elsewhere. It had shown (Figs. 10 and 11) right maxillary sinusitis with hyperdense foci with sclerosis and erosion of the maxillary sinus and inferior orbital wall with suspicion of fungal sinusitis and local invasion. Based on the scan, she had undergone nasal endoscopy elsewhere, and the tissue from the right maxillary sinus had shown Aspergillus species on KOH mount. So she had been started on oral voriconazole. A few weeks after voriconazole, due to

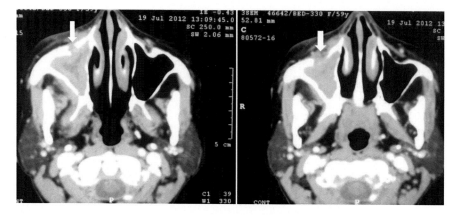

Fig. 11 Case 3: Axial CT contrast-enhanced scan shows the same lesion in the right maxillary sinus as in Fig. 10. Erosion is seen along the anterior wall of the right maxillary sinus (*arrows*)

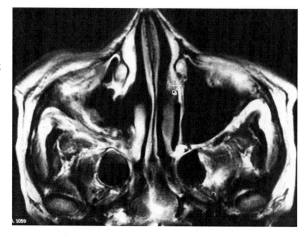

Fig. 12 Axial MRI scan showing decreased mucosal thickening and enhancement within the right maxillary with persistent ill-defined soft tissue and enhancement within the retro-maxillary fat

increasing severity of pain, she reported to us for a second opinion. On examination, nasal endoscopy showed only scarring from previous surgery.

Since no histopathological confirmation of the diagnosis of invasive fungal sinusitis was available from the first surgery, it was decided to obtain tissue for histopathology. MRI scan of the orbit and paranasal sinuses done at this time showed (Fig. 12) decrease in the mucosal thickening and enhancement within the right maxillary sinus and along the floor of the right orbit as compared to the previous CT scan. The ill-defined soft tissue and enhancement within the retro-maxillary fat extending into the infratemporal and pterygopalatine fossa were unchanged.

An endoscopic biopsy from the right medial maxillary wall as well as a subconjunctival biopsy from the infraorbital region was performed. On histopathology, the lesion showed moderately dense fibrosclerotic tissue with nodular and diffuse lymphoplasmacytic infiltrate. The lesion was seen eroding the bone, entrapping the vessels, nerves, and mucous glands. The entrapped glands were atrophic. There were no granulomas, no fungal infection, and no lymphoproliferative disorder. The lesion

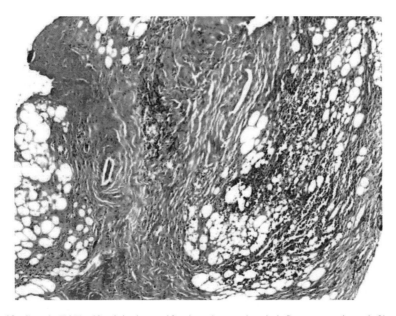

Fig. 13 Case 3: H&E ×40 original magnification: dense sclerotic inflammatory tissue infiltrating into fat

was diagnosed as inflammatory pseudotumor (Fig. 13) on histopathology. The patient was started on oral steroids and voriconazole was discontinued. Microbiology of the tissue was negative for fungus and bacteria. Voriconazole was discontinued, and patient was started on 40 mg oral steroids in divided doses. The patient was relieved of pain within a week of starting steroids. She has been symptom free for the past 5 months.

Discussion: Inflammatory pseudotumor (IPT) is a chronic, inflammatory, non-malignant lesion of unknown origin [12]. It is a space-occupying lesion produced by chronic inflammation and tissue fibrosis and is steroid responsive [13]. IPT in the head and neck region can be locally aggressive, with bony erosion and severe neuralgia like infraorbital neuralgia in this patient. Diagnosis is difficult as clinically and radiologically IPT is indistinguishable from invasive neoplasms [14–16] and invasive fungal lesions [17]. In this patient, it is debatable whether the initial treatment with oral voriconazole made it difficult to isolate *Aspergillus* spp. during the subsequent tissue sampling or whether the patient was a case of pseudotumor primarily who had been misdiagnosed as invasive Aspergillus sinusitis.

Case 4

A 45-year-old diabetic male came with an ulcer along the right nasolabial crease (Fig. 14) and a palatal ulcer (Fig. 15) since 3 months. It had been progressively increasing in size. Biopsy elsewhere had been inconclusive. Clinically it could be mistaken for invasive fungal sinusitis.

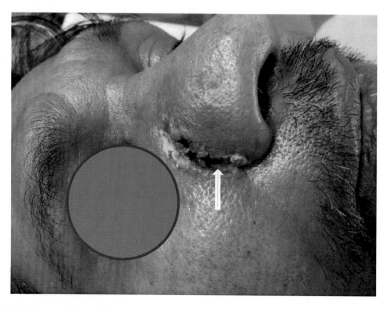

Fig. 14 Right nasolabial fold ulcer (*arrow*)

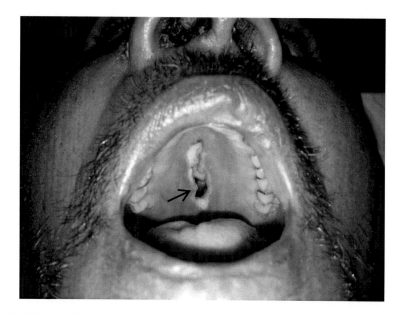

Fig. 15 Palatal perforation (*arrow*)

The biopsy was repeated, taking tissue from the palate. Histopathology revealed NK/T-cell lymphoma, and the patient was referred for chemotherapy – radiation.

Discussion: Clinically, the lesion could be mistaken for invasive fungal sinusitis, but histopathology is diagnostic and immunohistochemistry enables further

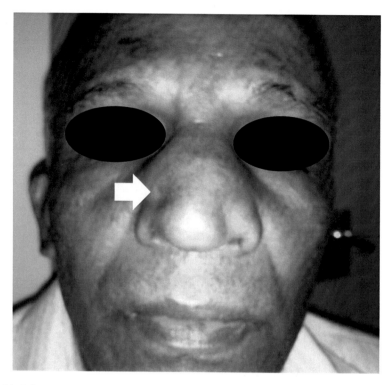

Fig. 16 Subcutaneous swelling (*arrow*) of the right nasal dorsum

classification of the tumor. In most cases EBV genomes are detectable in the tumor cells, and immunophenotyping may show CD56 positivity. NK/T-cell lymphoma is a rare, aggressive subtype of lymphoma associated with extensive necrosis and angioinvasion. It presents in extra-nodal regions, especially, the nasal or paranasal sinus region. Historically, this tumor was considered part of lethal midline granuloma. It may be associated with hemophagocytic syndrome and has a highly aggressive course with poor prognosis. In view of the poor response of the tumor to standard chemotherapy and radiation, some oncologists recommend bone marrow or peripheral stem cell transplantation.

Case 5

Mr M aged 55 complained of broadening of nose, nasal block, and occasional epistaxis since 5–6 months. On examination, the nose appeared broad (Fig. 16) (arrow) with thickening of the skin over the nasal dorsum. Anterior rhinoscopy showed hypertrophied turbinates, severe nasal mucosal congestion with no visible airway. Subcutaneous biopsy was obtained from the external nasal swelling. The biopsied tissue was sent for potassium hydroxide preparation and fungal culture. Broad thin-walled nonseptate mycelia were found in the KOH preparation. In the Sabouraud's dextrose agar medium are rapidly growing flat cream-colored colonies with conidia indicative of subcutaneous dermatomycoses or *Conidiobolus coronatus*. Patient was started on oral potassium iodide drops in tapering doses along with tab. fluconazole 200 mg daily. During treatment, the patient's thyroid function tests, SGPT, and serum potassium were monitored. The treatment was continued over 6 months, and the patient responded well with reduction in external nasal swelling. The nasal block disappeared, and the patient was able to breathe comfortably.

Discussion: Patients with rhinofacial swelling and unilateral nasal obstruction presenting to the ENT surgeon can present a diagnostic dilemma. Rhinoentomophthoromycosis (conidiobolomycosis) is a rare, chronic, localized, subcutaneous zygomycosis characterized by painless, woody swelling of the rhinofacial region [18]. Usually the lesion is firmly attached to the skin without involvement of the underlying bone. Therefore, tissue for testing has to be obtained from the affected subcutaneous tissue. It is a slowly progressive, but rarely life-threatening condition. It is caused by Conidiobolus coronatus (Entomophthora coronata), a fungus belonging to the order

Entomophthorales. KOH preparation of the biopsy tissue from the lesion reveals broad, nonseptate, thin-walled mycelial filaments. In Sabouraud's dextrose agar (SDA) medium, colonies of Conidiobolus coronatus grow rapidly. Histopathology shows fibroblastic proliferation, chronic granulomatous inflammatory reaction, and broad thin-walled hyphae [19].

Treatment of rhinoentomophthoromycosis is difficult because the diagnosis is delayed. Patients often respond to oral itraconazole (200–400 mg/day), ketoconazole (200–400 mg/day), fluconazole (100–200 mg/day), amphotericin B, and co-trimoxazole [20]. Prolonged treatment and follow-up is required.

Saturated potassium iodide solution (1 g/ml) is useful for patients because of its ease of administration and low cost.

References

Case 1

1. Schubert MS. Allergic fungal sinusitis: pathophysiology, diagnosis and management. Med Mycol. 2009;47(Suppl I):S324–30.
2. Stammberger H, Jaske R, Beaufort F. Aspergillosis of the paranasal sinus x-ray diagnosis, histopathology and clinical aspects. Ann Otol Rhinol Laryngol. 1984;93:251–6.
3. de Shazo RD, O'Brien M, Chapin K, Soto-Aguilar M, Gardner L, Swain R. A new classification and diagnostic criteria for invasive fungal sinusitis. Arch Otolaryngol Head Neck Surg. 1997;123:1181–8.
4. Gungor A, Adusumilli V, Corey JP. Fungal sinusitis progression of disease in immunosuppression – a case report. Ear Nose Throat J. 1998;77:207–15.
5. Seiberling K, Wormald PJ. The role of itraconazole in recalcitrant fungal sinusitis. Am J Rhinol Allergy. 2009;23(3):303–6. doi:10.2500/ajra.2009.23.3315.
6. Rains 3rd BM, Mineck CW. Treatment of allergic fungal sinusitis with high-dose itraconazole. Am J Rhinol. 2003;17(1):1–8.

Case 2

7. Grosjean P, Weber R. Fungus balls of the paranasal sinuses: a review. Eur Arch Otorhinolaryngol. 2007;264:461–70.
8. Dufour X, Kauffmann-Lacroix C, Ferrie JC, Goujon JM, Rodier MH, Klossek JM. Paranasal sinus fungal ball epidemiology, clinical features and diagnosis. A retrospective analysis of 173 cases from a single center in France: 1989–2002. Med Mycol. 2006;44:61–7.
9. de Shazo RD, O'Brien M, Chapin K, Soto-Aguilar M, Gardner L, Swain R. A new classification and diagnostic criteria for invasive fungal sinusitis. Arch Otolaryngol Head Neck Surg. 1997;123:1181–8.
10. Gungor A, Adusumilli V, Corey JP. Fungal sinusitis progression of disease in immunosuppression – a case report. Ear Nose Throat J. 1998;77:207–15.
11. Chakrabarti A, Denning DW, Ferguson BJ, et al. Fungal rhinosinusitis: a categorization and definitional schema addressing current controversies. Laryngoscope. 2009;119:1809–18.

Case 3

12. Som PM, Brandwein MS, Maldjian C, Reino AJ, Lawson W. Inflammatory pseudotumour of the maxillary sinus: CT and MR findings in six cases. AJR Am J Roentgenol. 1994;163(3):689–92.
13. Batsakis JG, Luna MA, el-Naggar AK, Goepfert H. Pathology consultation: inflammatory pseudotumour" – what is it? How does it behave? Ann Otol Rhinol Laryngol. 1995;104:329–31.
14. Han MH, Chi JG, Kim MS, Chang KH, Kim KH, Yeon KM, et al. Fibrosing inflammatory pseudotumours involving the skull base: MR and CT manifestations with histopathologic comparison. AJNR Am J Neuroradiol. 1996;17:515–21.
15. McKinney AM, Short J, Lucato L, Santacruz K, McKinney Z, Kim Y. Inflammatory myofibroblastic tumour of the orbit with associated enhancement of the meninges and multiple cranial nerves. AJNR Am J Neuroradiol. 2006;27:2217–20.
16. Chen JM, Moll C, Schotton JC, Fisch U. Inflammatory pseudotumours of the skull base. Skull Base Surg. 1994;4:93–8.
17. de Shazo RD, O'Brien M, Chapin K, Soto-Aguilar M, Gardner L, Swain R. A new classification and diagnostic criteria for invasive fungal sinusitis. Arch Otolaryngol Head Neck Surg. 1997;123:1181–8.

Case 5

18. Richardson MD, Warnock DW. Entomophromycosis. In: Richardson MD, Warnock DW, editors. Fungal infection. Diagnosis and management. 3rd ed. Chichester: Blackwell Publishing; 2003. p. 293–7.
19. Richardson MD, Pirkko KK, Gillian SS, et al. Rhizopus. Rhizomucor, absidia and other agents of systemic and subcutaneous zygomycosis. In: Patrick RM, Ellen JB, editors. Manual of clinical microbiology, vol. 2. 8th ed. Washington, DC: ASM Press; 2003. p. 1761–80.
20. Restrepo A. Treatment of tropical mycoses. J Am Acad Dermatol. 1994;31(3 Pt 2):S91–102.